Dennee Frey, PharmD
Editor

Improving Medication Management in Home Care: Issues and Solutions

Improving Medication Management in Home Care: Issues and Solutions has been co-published simultaneously as *Home Health Care Services Quarterly*, Volume 24, Numbers 1/2 2005.

Pre-publication REVIEWS, COMMENTARIES, EVALUATIONS . . .

"COMPREHENSIVE . . . INVALUABLE TO EVERYONE WORKING IN THE FIELD. Unlike so many publications that simply tell us how bad the problem is, this one shows us some of the proven ways to take action and improve care for our elderly patients. We all need to be thankful for The John A. Hartford Foundation's commitment to the field and editor Dennee Frey's talent for putting the results together in such a useful way."

Mark H. Beers, MD
Editor-in-Chief, *The Merck Manuals*

Improving Medication Management in Home Care: Issues and Solutions

Improving Medication Management in Home Care: Issues and Solutions has been co-published simultaneously as *Home Health Care Services Quarterly*, Volume 24, Numbers 1/2 2005.

Monographic Separates from *Home Health Care Services Quarterly*™

For additional information on these and other Haworth Press titles, including descriptions, tables of contents, reviews, and prices, use the QuickSearch catalog at http://www.HaworthPress.com.

Improving Medication Management in Home Care: Issues and Solutions, edited by Dennee Frey, PharmD (Vol. 24, No. 1/2, 2005). *A comprehensive examination of the issues and challenges faced in preventing medication errors with effective strategies for managing medication use in home and community care settings.*

A New Look at Community-Based Respite Programs: Utilization, Satisfaction, and Development, edited by Rhonda J.V. Montgomery, PhD (Vol. 21, No. 3/4, 2002). *"Clear, straightforward, and well focused on practical issues of service delivery . . . maintains a high standard of scholarship. A must-read for anyone interested in planning or evaluating respite services . . . . The first large-scale, longitudinal study of respite use. Service professionals, policymakers, and researchers in health policy, gerontology, and medical sociology will find the text of great value." (Judith G. Gonyea, PhD, Associate Professor, Boston University School of Social Work)*

The Next Generation of AIDS Patients: Service Needs and Vulnerabilities, edited by George J. Huba, PhD, Lisa A. Melchoir, PhD, A. T. Panter, PhD, Vivian B. Brown, PhD, David A. Cherin, PhD, and June Simmons, LCSW (Vol. 19, No. 1/2, 2001). *"Especially interesting in this volume is the presentation of an empirical model (CHAID) that both community-based organizations and service delivery systems can use to analyze client input to monitor and refine their HIV services." (Donna G. Anderson, PhD, MPH, Associate Professor, University of Colorado Health Sciences Center)*

AIDS Capitation, edited by David Alex Cherin, PhD, and G. J. Huba, PhD (Vol. 17, No. 1, 1998). *"A valuable resource to those interested in the blending of curative and palliative care and the application of this blended approach to catastrophic disease management." (Victor L. Kovner, MD, FACP, Medical Director, Sun Alliance Hospice)*

Personal Response Systems: An International Report of a New Home Care Service, edited by Andrew S. Dibner, PhD (Vol. 13, No. 3/4, 1993). *"Does a great service by reporting the forward strides taking place in other nations in the use of personal response systems (PRS)." (Daniel Thursz, DSW, ACSW, President, The National Council of Aging, Inc., Washington, DC)*

Facilitating Self Care Practices in the Elderly, edited by Barbara J. Horn, PhD, RN (Vol. 11, No. 1/2, 1990). *"Useful to researchers, practitioners, caregivers, and agencies providing care services to the elderly ill at home." (The Indian Journal of Social Work)*

Quality Impact of Home Care for the Elderly, edited by Francis G. Caro, PhD, and Arthur E. Blank, PhD (Vol. 9, No. 2/3, 1989). *"An excellent source of information for those wishing to increase their understanding of the home health care system or improve its effectiveness in their own community." (American Journal of Occupational Therapy)*

Worlds Apart?: Long-Term Care in Australia and the United States, edited by Sandra J. Newman, PhD (Vol. 8, No. 3, 1988). *An insightful comparison of how Australia and the United States are responding to the long-term care needs of the elderly.*

Health Care for the Elderly: Regional Responses for National Policy Issues, edited by Kathleen Gainor Andreoli, DSN, Leigh Anne Musser, MPH, and Stanley Joel Reiser, MD, PhD (Vol. 7, No. 3/4, 1987). *"One of the best, most comprehensive, and most penetratingly analytical works on elderly health care now available." (Health and Social Work)*

International Perspectives on Long-Term Care, edited by Laura Reif and Brahna Trager (Vol. 5, No. 3/4, 1985). *Experts from around the world address organizational and cost issues while offering innovative solutions for common problems in long-term care.*

Community-Based Systems of Long-Term Care, edited by Rick T. Zawadski, PhD (Vol. 4, No. 3/4, 1984). *Essential information on planning long-term health care services for the community.*

The Chronically Limited Elderly: The Case for a National Policy for In-Home and Supportive Community-Based Services, edited by Howard A. Palley, PhD, and Julianne S. Oktay, PhD (Vol. 4, No. 2, 1983). *"Compelling reading for those concerned about the non-institutional care of impaired elderly persons." (The Gerontologist)*

Family Home Care: Critical Issues for Services and Policies, edited by Robert Perlman, PhD (Vol. 3, No. 3/4, 1983). *"An important reference for those professionals working in the field of home health care." (Contemporary Sociology)*

Home Health Care and National Health Policy, edited by Brahna Trager (Vol. 1, No. 2, 1980). *A concise study of the current status of home health care in the United States.*

Improving Medication Management in Home Care: Issues and Solutions

Dennee Frey, PharmD
Editor

Improving Medication Management in Home Care: Issues and Solutions has been co-published simultaneously as *Home Health Care Services Quarterly*, Volume 24, Numbers 1/2 2005.

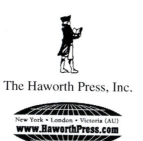

The Haworth Press, Inc.

New York • London • Victoria (AU)
www.HaworthPress.com

Improving Medication Management in Home Care: Issues and Solutions has been co-published simultaneously as *Home Health Care Services Quarterly*™, Volume 24, Numbers 1/2 2005.

The development, preparation, and publication of this work has been undertaken with great care. However, the publisher, employees, editors, and agents of The Haworth Press and all imprints of The Haworth Press, Inc., including The Haworth Medical Press® and Pharmaceutical Products Press®, are not responsible for any errors contained herein or for consequences that may ensue from use of materials or information contained in this work. Opinions expressed by the author(s) are not necessarily those of The Haworth Press, Inc. With regard to case studies, identities and circumstances of individuals discussed herein have been changed to protect confidentiality. Any resemblance to actual persons, living or dead, is entirely coincidental.

The Haworth Press, Inc., 10 Alice Street, Binghamton, NY 73904-1580 USA

Cover design by Kerry Mack

Library of Congress Cataloging-in-Publication Data

Improving medication management in home care: issues and solutions / Dennee Frey, editor.
　　p. cm.
　　"Co-published simultaneously as Home Health Care Services Quarterly, Volume 24, Numbers 1/2, 2005."
　　Includes bibliographical references and index.
　　ISBN-10: 0-7890-3052-7 (hard cover : alk. paper)
　　ISBN-13: 978-0-7890-3052-8 (hard cover : alk. paper)
　　ISBN-10: 0-7890-3053-5 (soft cover : alk. paper)
　　ISBN-13: 978-0-7890-3053-5 (soft cover : alk. paper)
　　1. Geriatric pharmacology. 2. Medication errors–Prevention. 3. Older people–Drug use.
　4. Older people–Home care. 5. Home care services–Quality control.
　　[DNLM: 1. Home Care Services. 2. Medication Errors–prevention & control. W Y 115 I348
2005] I. Frey, Dennee.
　RC953.7.I53 2005
　615.5'8'0846–dc22
                                                                                    2005013428

Indexing, Abstracting & Website/Internet Coverage

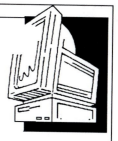

This section provides you with a list of major indexing & abstracting services and other tools for bibliographic access. That is to say, each service began covering this periodical during the year noted in the right column. Most Websites which are listed below have indicated that they will either post, disseminate, compile, archive, cite or alert their own Website users with research-based content from this work. (This list is as current as the copyright date of this publication.)

Abstracting, Website/Indexing Coverage . . . . Year When Coverage Began

- *Abstracts in Social Gerontology: Current Literature on Aging* **1989**
- *AgeInfo CD-ROM <http://www.cpa.org.uk>* **1995**
- *AgeLine Database <http://www.research.aarp.org/ageline>* **1979**
- *AGRICOLA Database (AGRICultural OnLine Access)*
  A Bibliographic database of citations to the agricultural literature created by the National Agricultural Library and its cooperators <http://www.natl.usda.gov/ag98> **1994**
- *AGRIS <http://www.fao.org/agris/>* **1994**
- *Alzheimer's Disease Education & Referral Center (ADEAR)* **1995**
- *Business Source Corporate: coverage of nearly 3,350 quality magazines and journals; designed to meet the diverse information needs of corporations; EBSCO Publishing <http://www.epnet.com/corporate/bsourcecorp.asp>* **2003**
- *Cambridge Scientific Abstracts is a leading publisher of scientific information in print journals, online databases, CD-ROM and via the Internet <http://www.csa.com>* **1991**

(continued)

(continued)

* **Exact start date to come**

(continued)

*Special Bibliographic Notes related to special journal issues
(separates) and indexing/abstracting:*

- indexing/abstracting services in this list will also cover material in any "separate" that is co-published simultaneously with Haworth's special thematic journal issue or DocuSerial. Indexing/abstracting usually covers material at the article/chapter level.
- monographic co-editions are intended for either non-subscribers or libraries which intend to purchase a second copy for their circulating collections.
- monographic co-editions are reported to all jobbers/wholesalers/approval plans. The source journal is listed as the "series" to assist the prevention of duplicate purchasing in the same manner utilized for books-in-series.
- to facilitate user/access services all indexing/abstracting services are encouraged to utilize the co-indexing entry note indicated at the bottom of the first page of each article/chapter/contribution.
- this is intended to assist a library user of any reference tool (whether print, electronic, online, or CD-ROM) to locate the monographic version if the library has purchased this version but not a subscription to the source journal.
- individual articles/chapters in any Haworth publication are also available through the Haworth Document Delivery Service (HDDS).

ABOUT THE EDITOR

Dennee Frey, PharmD, has over 20 years experience in home care and long-term care, including as a consultant pharmacist working directly with clinicians at the former Visiting Nurse Association of Los Angeles. She has developed and implemented several national, multi-site demonstration projects in geriatric, HIV/AIDS and Hospice/palliative home care; has served as Consultant Pharmacist/Project Director for VNA-LA and Field Consultant for JCAHO Home Health Program; has been an active member of the American Society of Consultant Pharmacists; has participated in the Editorial Review Board of *Home Health Care Services Quarterly*; and has presented at local, state and national home care and pharmacy associations on a variety of topics. Since 1985, Dr. Frey has had an appointment as Adjunct Assistant Professor of Clinical Pharmacy at the University of Southern California, School of Pharmacy. She currently serves as Consultant Pharmacist/Project Director of the *Medications Management Model* for identification and reduction of medication errors in care management sites. This project is one of 13 in the national Administration on Aging Evidence-Based Prevention Initiative. Dr. Frey is committed to improving medication management and advancing the practice of consultant pharmacists in home health and long-term care.

Improving Medication Management in Home Care: Issues and Solutions

CONTENTS

Preface:
Bringing New Evidence-Based Tools
to Strengthen Practice

This Special Volume focuses on the important area of medications management–the identification of errors and the development of cost-effective models to improve this key area of clinical practice. Partners in Care Foundation, has worked on the issue of medication errors for many years, beginning with work conducted under Visiting Nurse Association of Los Angeles, continuing through the past seven years under Partners in Care Foundation. We have discovered what the literature now confirms–that medication errors occur with a shocking frequency. Improving medication management represents an area for healthcare quality improvement and a symptom of concern that requires healthcare reform.

Partners in Care Foundation was formed to "change the shape of healthcare," especially in home and community care settings. We work to identify problems of magnitude in which large populations are negatively impacted, even though major financial investments are already funneled to these areas through healthcare dollars. Under this definition, it's easy to see why we have made medications management a major priority.

The original medication errors work focused on the home health care arena where we worked with Vanderbilt University to develop a Medications Management Model. The study identified high prevalence rates of medications errors in the Medicare population receiving skilled home health services, and a successful intervention to improve medication management was developed to address this problem. Results of this work revealed that through proper screening for errors coupled with the services of a consulting clinical pharmacist, we can significantly reduce

[Haworth co-indexing entry note]: "Preface: Bringing New Evidence-Based Tools to Strengthen Practice." Simmons, W. June. Co-published simultaneously in *Home Health Care Services Quarterly* (The Haworth Press, Inc.) Vol. 24, No. 1/2, 2005, pp. xxi-xxv; and: *Improving Medication Management in Home Care: Issues and Solutions* (ed: Dennee Frey) The Haworth Press, Inc., 2005, pp. xv-xix. Single or multiple copies of this article are available for a fee from The Haworth Document Delivery Service [1-800- HAWORTH, 9:00 a.m. - 5:00 p.m. (EST). E-mail address: docdelivery@haworthpress.com].

Available online at http://www.haworthpress.com/web/HHC

those errors. The older home health population, who frequently has medical co-morbidities treated by multiple physicians and frequent interactions with a variety of specializations, was caught in the dilemma of a fragmented healthcare system; there is limited reimbursement for coordination of care between physicians, and it is a role which has not been assigned to any one physician. As a result, it is easy to have drug duplication and/or interactions which can harm patients and even lead to death. With ongoing support from the John A. Hartford Foundation, Partners in Care Foundation undertook an effort to disseminate the Vanderbilt University Medications Management Model findings to home health providers nationwide.

Several agencies' experiences in translating research into practice are described in this Special Collection. The successful demonstration of the effectiveness of focusing quality improvement in these clinical settings was encouraging and led us to pursue this work in other arenas. Of particular interest are programs in which staff is currently mandated to review medications and assess their use (over and under) and place this data in the medical record. Here we see that our healthcare dollar already pays for the labor to capture the information from which a coordinated review of all medications can occur. Yet, unlike the nursing home where pharmacy review is required, home health and other home care programs are not under mandatory pharmacy review. Home health agencies in fact have no specific mechanism to pay for such reviews under their reimbursement formulas.

Looking beyond home health agencies, we noted that Medicaid Waivers for frail dually eligible Medicaid and Medicare elderly target this high-risk population as well. The dually eligible represent about 16% of the over 65 population and are high utilizers who consume about one-third of all Medicare health resources. Of this population, nearly 1,000,000 nationwide are enrolled in state directed Medicaid waiver programs which target nursing home certified frail elderly in order to help them remain at home. Here they receive care management support from nurse/social work teams coupled with a benefit allowing the purchase of "waived" services in order to support their ability to remain at home and avoid nursing home placement. This is different from home health in which clients receive skilled medical care and supervision in the home under MD orders.

The Waiver programs are much more focused on coordination of all needs with a strong emphasis on independent functioning and services which compensate for a loss of these abilities in order to assure safe, independent living in the community. Thus Medicaid Waiver programs are not medical programs, but rather are programs that focus on service coordination including assuring timely access to needed medical services. These programs are hybrid social-medical models of care management that serve large numbers of individuals and do so for a longer period of time than home health is usually permitted under current home health regulation and design, especially since the introduction of home health payment per episode of care (prospective payment). The structure of this model includes periodic medication inventory, and, as such, provides an opportunity for identifying and eliminating medication errors.

This Special Volume reports findings and lessons learned from the work of many, focusing on broad epidemiological reviews of medication coordination issues as well as the specific focus on home health as an arena of care. In this Preface, I wish to point to the emerging work now underway through Partners in Care Foundation and our clinical partners at Senior Care Network of Huntington Hospital in Pasadena, California. After the very successful efforts and results of our medications work in the home health arena, we became interested in whether or not the same kind of approach could be adapted to identify and resolve medications errors in Medicaid Waivers designed to target frail elders at risk of nursing home placement, as discussed above.

We were successful in bringing the Medication Management Model that evolved from the Vanderbilt University study to the testing stage through support from the Administration on Aging (AoA) Evidence-Based Prevention Initiative (EBPI). It was proposed that we identify prevalence rates and pilot the role of the consulting pharmacist in medication management in the California Medicaid Waiver, the Multi-Purpose Senior Services Program known colloquially as MSSP. This statewide program serves nearly 12,000 frail dually eligible seniors on any given day through 41 sites throughout the state. It is similar to programs sponsored by most states that serve, in total, over 900,000 such individuals nationally. The development of a cost-effective approach to medications in these settings has great potential to improve health-status with the development and introduction of a simple method of screening in high-risk cases and providing pharmacist review of problem cases.

MSSPCare is a software that supports an integrated electronic medical record and billing system for MSSP sites. This software was developed by RTZ, a software company in northern California with a strategic focus on coordination of services for frail older adults. It is currently in use in 14 sites throughout the state. Our AoA EBPI medication management program led by Dennee Frey, PharmD, the editor of this volume, is partnering with RTZ to add a medications listing and screening component to this electronic system. This system is designed to identify clients at risk of medication error for pharmacist review through a computerized risk assessment screening. The program is in early stages of design and testing, but early results are encouraging. The software algorithm and intervention protocols build on our prior work with Vanderbilt, under the guidance of a geriatric advisory panel. In addition, although computerized screening is more efficient and cost effective, paper screening approaches are being used as well; because many settings do not have the ability or will to adopt an electronic system to support this program.

One of the areas of success appears to be staff acceptance of the importance and feasibility of this new tool for their practice. Often the introduction of innovation in clinical settings is challenging–clinicians are extremely busy and new approaches are time-intensive, so there can be resistance to change. Our early experience in medication management in these non-medical programs suggests a welcoming practice environment as the need for this type of intervention is recognized. The clients' medical conditions are complex and their medication use is high. The risk of errors is great, and the availability of medical coordination very limited.

In fact staff identified the need for improvement in this area. Care management staff, social workers and nurses alike, have been very motivated as they are aware that medication errors, short of increasing mortality rates, often lead to avoidable confusion, dizziness and high risk of falls. Falls prevention, in particular, seems a shared concern of all as falls can represent a tipping point and pose great risk of injury, thus threatening both patient safety and the continued ability to live independently. In addition, since staff are already required to collect all the medications for the medical record, the added labor for this powerful intervention is minimal. This, of course, helps make it a practical innovation.

Early screenings during the pilot stages of this program indicate that medication errors may be even higher in this population than in the home health population. This might be in part because the program does not require physician orders as home health does. Therefore it is not surprising that elderly with complex co-morbidities, functional losses but much more limited medical coordination of their care potentially have a higher rate of medication errors. Our AoA project will provide prevalency rates as well as data on the effectiveness of this model in the two programs in which the intervention is being tested. If, as suspected, a much higher error rate is occurring, the opportunity for improvement is therefore extremely significant.

America invests huge resources in healthcare and invests heavily in the Waiver programs in an effort to support independent living, an approach even more important in light of the Olmstead ruling mandating choice for the frail elder. By federal mandate skilled nursing facilities require that pharmacist consultation be provided to each patient on a routine basis. No such mandate exists in the care management setting to protect Medicaid-Waiver clients, although they are just as needy and frail as institutionalized patients. It seems clear that powerful new tools to support their vital work will have great strategic value through improving the clinical results from the program investments already in place. Strengthening these efforts through introduction of evidence-based innovations is a high priority for Partners in Care Foundation as well as with our nation's health care leaders. This work continues to unfold in Partners' effort to change the shape of healthcare for the better.

W. June Simmons, LCSW
Editor
Home Health Care Services Quarterly

Acknowledgment

This volume was supported in part by grant funding from the The John A. Hartford Foundation, Inc., New York, New York, a non-profit grant-making organization that funds programs that aim to integrate and improve health services for older adults. The Foundation awarded funding to Partners in Care Foundation to disseminate the Medication Management Model program to home health providers and facilitate its adoption into everyday agency practice. On-site technical assistance was provided by Partners to four leading home health providers across the country. The Medication Management Model is based on a previously successful demonstration project that improved medication use and reduced medication errors among elderly home health patients. Project results and materials can be found at *www.homemeds.org*. Click on Preventing Medication Errors: The Home Health Medication Model.

Partners in Care Foundation is a Los Angeles County-based non-profit organization that assists health care providers and community-based organizations to create, implement and evaluate new ways of delivering care.

Introduction

Dennee Frey, PharmD

Much has been written about the issue of medication use in the elderly over the last two decades.[4,15,18] Older adults are at especially high risk for medication errors and medication-related problems due to biological changes associated with aging and disease[8] coupled with their heavy use of medications–an average of six a day. A 1998 report in the *Journal of the American Medication Association* noted that medication errors had become so widespread among the elderly that if they were classified as a distinct disease they would rank as the fifth-leading cause of death for Americans over age 65.[6] In fact, it is estimated that medication errors claim one life every 71 minutes.[18] Furthermore, in 2002, the United States spent $177 billion on treating medication-related errors.[13]

The problems that arise from medication misuse in various settings from hospital to the community are well documented.[5,8,10,11,12,14,17,19,22,23] In recent years since the publication of the landmark Institute of Medicine report, *To Err Is Human*, more attention is being focused on this issue by policymakers, institutions and clinicians.[1,18] Priority is being given to strategies for reducing medication errors and improving the quality of care at all levels. Hospitals are using information technology to reduce rates of medication errors and improve care coordination. Clinically, there is increased emphasis on evidence-based medicine and rational prescribing of medications, particularly in the aging population, to maximize clinical benefit and minimize adverse events such as medication-related problems. Patient safety and other standards on an

---

[Haworth co-indexing entry note]: "Introduction." Frey, Dennee. Co-published simultaneously in *Home Health Care Services Quarterly* (The Haworth Press, Inc.) Vol. 24, No. 1/2, 2005, pp. 1-11; and: *Improving Medication Management in Home Care: Issues and Solutions* (ed: Dennee Frey) The Haworth Press, Inc., 2005, pp. 1-11. Single or multiple copies of this article are available for a fee from The Haworth Document Delivery Service [1-800-HAWORTH, 9:00 a.m. - 5:00 p.m. (EST). E-mail address: docdelivery@haworth press.com].

Available online at http://www.haworthpress.com/web/HHC
doi:10.1300/J027v24n01_01

individual care level implemented by accrediting agencies such as the Joint Commission on Accreditation of Health Care Organizations seek to improve medication management.[24]

There is a particular need to improve the systematic management of medication for community-dwelling older adults as this population ages and continues to live independently in the community. Recent findings indicate that inappropriate medication use by community-dwelling elders ranges from 12-40%. Frail elders, particularly those who are homebound, may be even more vulnerable to medication-related problems for a variety of reasons such as co-morbid chronic conditions and socio-economic factors.[23]

The articles included in this volume all address issues of medication management in home care settings as well as transitional care from the hospital back to the community. Areas of opportunity for improvement, successful model interventions and pilot programs are discussed as are challenges faced in implementing these interventions on a program level, and barriers to successful and sustained progress. Solutions put forward by the authors for improving medication management include systematic approaches such as developing computerized risk assessment screenings, implementing pharmacist-centered interventions, improving transitional care and strengthening the interdisciplinary team. Recommendations for further research to demonstrate benefits of these interventions are presented as well.

An emphasis on pharmacist-centered interventions in this issue is especially relevant for several reasons. In 2003, improving medication management was identified as a national priority by the National Institute of Medicine (NIM) in a report that also underscored the important role pharmacists play in monitoring patients' drug therapies. The report calls for greater involvement of pharmacists in patient care to help prevent medication-related problems.[1] The second reason is the implementation in 2006 of Part D of the Medicare Modernization Act (MMA) of 2003. This is a provision that high-risk or "targeted" beneficiaries receive Medication Therapy Management (MTM) Services and provides potential funding for pharmacist interventions. The final reason is the impetus for this special publication, to disseminate the results of adapting a tested pharmacist-centered medication management intervention into home health agencies across the country.

The first set of articles report on the experience of adapting this evidence-based medication management model (MMM) into everyday agency practice. As background, in 1997 two of the nation's largest home health agencies at the time–the Visiting Nurse Association of Los

Angeles (VNA-LA) and Visiting Nurse Service New York (VNS-NY)– joined researchers at Vanderbilt University Department of Preventive Medicine to develop and test a model of care to improve pharmacotherapy in home health patients.[9] A consensus panel of experts was convened and identified these target evidence-based high-risk problems: unnecessary therapeutic duplication; cardiovascular medication problems; use of psychotropic drugs in patients with a reported recent fall or confusion; and use of non-steroidal anti-inflammatory drugs (NSAIDs) in high-risk patients.

The first phase of the study, to determine the incidence of potential medication errors in their elderly Medicare patients, found that the proportion of patients at risk of medication errors was high: up to 30% of the 6,718 home health patients in the study had a possible error according to Home Health criteria developed for the study and the well-established Beers criteria. The potential error rate increased with the number of medications taken.[9]

The next phase of the study was a randomized controlled trial that tested a pharmacist intervention to improve medication use in patients identified at high risk with the Home Health Criteria. The intervention consisted of advice from a consultant pharmacist to home health staff based on clinical guidelines developed for the project. Medication use improved significantly in 50% of intervention patients, compared to 38% of controls (p = .05). Improvement was greatest for interventions with therapeutic duplication and cardiovascular problems.[21]

Due to the significant findings of this intervention, The John A. Hartford Foundation, Inc., the study's funder, supported an additional technical assistance/dissemination phase to facilitate adaptation of what is now the Medication Management Model (MMM) into everyday practice by other home health agencies The Foundation funded Partners in Care Foundation (Partners) to disseminate study findings through a website <www.homemeds.org>, created to provide a toolkit of materials essential to agencies wishing to adapt the model, and to provide technical assistance consultation to agencies interested in adapting the model of care.

Additionally on-site technical assistance was provided by Partners to four home health agencies across the country to adapt the MMM into their agency practice and to learn from their experiences. The four agencies were the Visiting Nurse Service, New York City; Home Care Plus, Lewisburg, West Virginia; the Eddy Visiting Nurse Association, Catskill, New York branch and Memorial Care Home Health Agency, Long Beach, California.

Each of the agencies had a common goal: to improve medication management and prevent medication-related problems in their elderly clients residing at home. Each applied the model in a singular way, particular to that agency. The sites were chosen to reflect the continuum of home health service providers across the country: from urban to rural; for-profit and not for profit; sole proprietary to a branch of a regional healthcare system; small to monolithic. Site profiles and adaptation materials are available at <www.homemeds.org>.

The VNS New York Congregate Care program was the initial technical assistance site and was instrumental in adapting processes from the original study that the other three technical assistance sites then followed. Established in the 1980s, the program includes congregate settings such as Senior Housing, Natural Occurring Retirement Communities (NORCs), public housing, Single Room Occupancy (SRO) hotels and private apartment buildings and complexes. The program's goal is to promote successful community living by strengthening collaboration between residents, building/facility management, building lay-leadership and the health care agency. Health education, health promotion, health screening, health linkages and direct service provision are provided on-site for building residents. Each congregate site represents its own unique culture.

This site focused medication management services on patients living in naturally occurring retirement centers (NORC) in Manhattan. Consultant services were provided by a contract pharmacist contracted on an hourly basis. The site developed a screening process that included a manual "Trigger Tool" to identify patients at highest risk. The process, along with the medication section of the automated Plan of Care available to staff on their portable computer tablet, allows the nurse to problem-solve medication issues and work with the pharmacist and physician to prevent medication errors in the home-based care environments. The agency concluded that the MMM intervention can make the difference between a resident successfully managing their health or experiencing a decline of functioning that can lead to hospitalization or long term institutional care.[16]

In the other three technical sites the medication management model also proved to be feasible, versatile and sustainable as described in the articles included in this volume. Each of the sites implemented the MMM within the agency's continuous quality improvement (CQI) activities, usually as part of an accreditation process. Along the way we learned at large, urban, hospital-based Memorial Care Home Health that the medication management model can help expand a home health agency's ability to prevent falls, a performance improvement indicator; at the smaller, rural, free-standing and proprietary Home Care Plus that the MMM can be successfully implemented and integrated with other assessment processes; and at the rural branch of the Eddy VNA that the MMM can provide a framework by which faculty pharmacist and intern pharmacists can cost-effectively provide pharmaceutical care services to improve care to home health waiver clients.

Overall the technical assistance phase yielded key elements of program adaptation and numerous lessons learned as well as future directions for providing pharmacist-centered interventions in other community-based programs. Among these was the possible application of the Model in other home and community care programs, particularly care management waiver programs. Partners currently is conducting model adaptation work in a population of dually-eligible frail elders receiving waiver services from California's Multi-purpose Senior Services Program (MSSP). The project is funded by the U.S. Dept. of Health and Human Services Administration on Aging as part of their Evidence-Based Prevention Program for the Elderly. This initiative is a public/private partnership to increase access for older people to programs that have proven to be effective in reducing the risk of disease, injury, and disability to help implement evidence-based prevention programs through aging services providers at the community level. The areas of focus include medication management as well as falls prevention, disease self-management, nutrition, and physical activity. Partners study is producing extensive knowledge about integrating the model and its consultant pharmacist intervention in the care management programs and factors in translating research into practice. Findings will be reported in an upcoming issue of this journal.

The first three articles in this volume describe how the home health agencies participating in Partner's technical assistance work applied the MMM to programs within their organizations. From their experience we hope readers will be able to gain insight into the value of adapting this pharmacist-centered intervention and the importance of integrating the model with other assessment processes.

"A Quality Improvement Project to Reduce Falls and Improve Medication Management," by authors Sperling, Neal, Hales, Adams, and Frey, discusses implementing the Model as part of a medical center's overall CQI program to improve falls prevention. The article describes the experience of the technical assistance site Memorial Home Health Care, a division of Long Beach Memorial Medical Center, and may be especially timely because it addresses application of recent accreditation medication management and patient safety standards. Among the lessons learned was the value of the model in assessing and reporting falls and that a positive interaction took place between patients and the pharmacist.

In "Integration of a Medication Management Model into Outcome-Based Quality Improvement: A Pilot Program in a Rural Proprietary Home Healthcare Agency," Atkinson and Frey discuss integrating the model's intervention with mandated patient care assessment data, the OASIS, through a computerized medication risk screening process piloted at Home Care Plus. The process described has the potential to help other home care providers maximize resources and decrease burden on staff. It is the authors' opinion that this process moves the pharmacist intervention from a focused drug regimen review to medication therapy management, and that this has potential reimbursement implications with implementation of Part D of the Medicare Drug Act in 2006.

The collaboration between a home heath care agency and a college of pharmacy to adapt the model and provide a cost-effective intervention in an under-served rural area is explored in Triller's "Medication Management Model as Experiential Education Tool for Students of Pharmacy." A pharmaceutical care service using intern pharmacists was implemented by the Eddy VNA's Catskill branch in their care management waiver program. It proved to be a successful and mutually beneficial arrangement that can be considered by other providers with near-by pharmacy clerkship programs and provides a framework for clinical pharmacist services to high-risk patients identified through an agency's CQI process.

Home care includes in-home services such as care management programs for frail community-dwelling elderly, a population potentially at highest risk for medication related problems. Williams and Lopez discuss this important issue and illustrate another model of pharmacist intervention in their article "Reaching the Homebound Elderly: The Prescription Intervention and Lifelong Learning (PILL) Program" that describes a recent three-year pilot project to develop in-home pharmacy care services to clients of a community-based social service agency. They found that agency clients were highly vulnerable to medication-related problems and were in need of in-home pharmacy care services. The question of on-going funding to sustain successful intervention was raised.

Reimbursement of medication management services is the topic of "Comment on Medication Management Models and Other Pharmacist Interventions: Implications for Policy and Practice" by Cameron. Implementation of the Medicare Modernization Act (MMA) of 2003 poses challenges for policy makers and administrators, including a provision that high-risk or "targeted" beneficiaries receive Medication Therapy Management (MTM) Services. These services are part of Medicare Part D and go into effect in January 2006. The article comments on the policy and practice implications of providing MTM, including recommendations of the American Society of Consultant Pharmacists (ASCP) and presents the Medication Management Model and other community-based pharmacist-centered interventions as examples of solutions to improve medication management and prevent medication-related problems in Medicare beneficiaries.

In "Polypharmacy and Possible Drug-Drug Interactions Among Diabetic Patients Receiving Home Health Care Services," Ibrahim, Kang, and Dansky, examine the prevalence of polypharmacy and possible drug-drug interactions in diabetic patients receiving home health care services, They report findings on the degree of potential significant interactions and suggestions for systematic monitoring to identify polypharmacy in patients with chronic co-morbid conditions such as diabetes. Among their conclusions is the need for systematic monitoring of drug regimens and that home health care takers are in a position to identify polypharmacy and to modify drug regimens.

The article "Opportunities for Improving Post-Hospital Home Medication Management Among Older Adults," Foust, Naylor, Boling, and Cappuzzo thoroughly explores this issue using Reason's human error theory to frame the discussion of complex, system-oriented factors that inadvertently affect post-hospital medication problems. Post-hospital adverse drug events and medication-related risk factors are reviewed to describe high-risk older adults as a population that may most likely benefit from targeted interventions. Potential solutions and directions for future research highlight the importance of interdisciplinary teams, involvement of clinical pharmacists, use of transitional care and informational technologies.

Enguidanos and Brumley provide a real-life example of the challenges in improving the system via technology in "Risk of Medication Errors at Hospital Discharge and Barriers to Problem Resolution." They conducted a pilot to identify medication documentation problems at the point of hospital discharge. The article discusses the difficulties encountered in developing new technological processes as well as patient and physician attitudes about the medications communication efforts.

In the culminating article, "Medications Management in Older Persons: What Can Be Achieved by the International Community?" Azzopardi reminds us of the universal nature of all of the medication issues previously discussed. Improved drug prescribing through rational drug use, interdisciplinary medication management and systematic drug review are some considerations being promoted in the international community. The author comments on these and other issues presented at a recent conference sponsored by the United Nation's International Institute on Aging-Malta and other European organizations. An important conclusion raised by the European Director of the World Health Organization is that once patients get their medications–either post discharge from the hospital or after visiting a practitioner–little is known about what happens at home. He advocates that more resources need to be allocated for management in this area.

An innovative model of government-funded in-home medication services that came to our attention during the conference is one funded by the Australian Department of Health and Aging. They have implemented an integrative service that utilizes an interdisciplinary team of general practitioner and pharmacist with a patient-focused medication management approach. Studies conducted in Australia have found that programs with this service had positive clinical results, including understanding of and concordance with medication regimens and improved patient satisfaction, and had a significant reduction in healthcare costs.[3] This model may have implications in our own country as we move forward with federally-funded Medication Management Therapy Services and has particular relevance to the theme of this collection.

ACKNOWLEDGMENTS

The impetus for this volume was the Medication Management Model dissemination and technical assistance phase previously mentioned and funded by the John A. Hartford Foundation, Inc., New York, New York. We extend our sincere gratitude to the Foundation for their support, particularly to project officers Christopher Langston, PhD, and Sarahjane Bettis, PhD, for their judicious oversight; and to Foundation consultants JoAnne Handy, RN, MS, for her expert and insightful site visit consultation and Mark Beers, MD, for his strategic leadership and thoughtful evaluation of the project's results. The research team at Vanderbilt University Department of Preventive Medicine, including Principal Investigator Wayne Ray, PhD, and Project Director Sarah Meredith, who developed the seminal study on which our work was built, provided valuable consultation. Particular thanks to their associate Kathi Hall for developing the computer risk assessment algorithm and assistance in implementation at Home Care Plus.

This demonstration project has been one of successful collaboration on so many levels. I want to thank in particular the administrators, staff and managers of each of the four technical assistance sites for their commitment to improving patient care and vision in implementing this project, particularly the Visiting Nurse Service of New York's Congregate Care Program which was the inaugural MMM technical assistance site. They worked diligently to develop and test the initial trigger tool and procedures adopted and refined by the three sites that followed.

Further thanks are in order: To Annie Rahman, MSW, for her assistance with manuscript preparation and website content and editing; To the Project Advisory Committee, Karen Crockett Lindstrom, PT, MBA, Joan Marren, RN, Penny Feldman, PhD, Peter Boling, MD, Bradley Williams, PharmD, for their guidance and expertise, and also to Corridor Group principals Jeanne Parker Martin, RN, MPH, and Heidi O'Connor, MA, for their support and assistance in site selection; To Partners in Care Foundation's Communication Team, including the Director of Strategic Communications, Jody Dunn, and webmaster J. Frederick Helmut 2002 Colours for website development and maintenance. Finally I want to acknowledge the contributions and energetic efforts of the MMM team Mira Trufasiu, Jennifer Wieckowski, and Nancy Vong, without whom this volume would not have been possible.

REFERENCES

1. Adams, K., and Corrigan, J.M. (Eds.) (2003). *Priority areas for quality improvement: Transforming health care quality.* National Academies' Institute of Medicine. 41-114.

2. Administration on Aging (AoA). (n.d.). *Evidence-based prevention program for the elderly.* Retrieved on January 15, 2005 from http://www.aoa.gov.

3. Australian Government Department is Health and Aging. (2004, August 24). *Home Medicines Review (HMR) Guidelines.* Retrieved December 10, 2004 from http://www.health.gov.au/internet/wcms/publishing.nsf/Content/health-epc-dmmr.htm.

4. Barker, K.N., Flynn, E.A., Pepper, G.A., Bates, D.W., & Mikeal, R.L. (2002). Medication errors observed in 36 health care facilities. *Archives Internal Medicine, 162,* 1897-1903.

5. Bates, D.W. (2000). Using information technology to reduce rates of medication errors in hospitals. *British Medical Journal, 320,* 788-791.

6. Bates, D.W. (1997). The costs of adverse drug events in hospitalized patients. *Journal of the American Medical Association, 277,* 307-311.

7. Bates, D.W., Cullen, D. J., Laird, N., Peterson, L. A., Small, S. D., & Servi, D. (1995). Incidence of adverse drug events and potential adverse drug events: Implications for prevention. *JAMA, 274*(1), 29-34.

8. Beers, M. H. (2001). Age-related changes as a risk factor for medication-related problems. *Generations, 4*, 22-27.

9. Brown, N.J., Griffin, M.R., Ray, W.A., Meredith, S., Beers, M.H., Marren, J., Robles, M., Stergachis, A., Wood, A.J.J., & Avorn, J. (1998). A model for improving medication use in home health care patients. *Journal Am Pharm Association, 38*:696-702.

10. Boockvar, K., Fishman, E., Kyriacou, C.K., Monias, A., Gavi, S., & Cortes, T. (2004). Adverse events due to discontinuations in drug use and dose changes in patients transferred between acute and long-term care facilities. *Arch Intern Med, 164*(5), 545-550.

11. Col, N., Fanale, J.E., & Kronholm, P. (1990) The role of medication noncompliance and adverse drug reactions in hospitalization of the elderly. *Arch Intern Med, 150*(4), 841-845.

12. Curtis, L. H., Østbye, T., Sendersky, V. et al. (2004). Inappropriate prescribing for elderly Americans in a large outpatient population. *Arch Intern Med, 164*(15), 1621-1625.

13. Ernst, F., & Grizzle, A. (2001). Drug related morbidity and mortality: Updating the cost-of-illness model. *Journal Am Pharm Association, 41*, 192-199.

14. Flaherty, J.H., Perry, H.M., & Lynchard, G.S. et al. (2000) Polypharmacy and hospitalization among older home care patients. *J Gerontol: Med Sci, 55A* (10), M554-M559.

15. Food and Drug Administration (FDA). (n.d.) Retrieved on January 12, 2005 from http://www.fda.org.

16. Hawkey, R. (2003). *VNS final report*. Unpublished report for the Visiting Nurse Service New York, NY.

17. Hanlon, J.T., Artz, M.B., Pieper, C.F., Lindblad, C.I., Sloane, R.J., Ruby, C.M., & Schmader, K.E. (2004). Inappropriate medication use among frail elderly inpatients. *Annals of Pharmacotherapy, 38*(1), 9-14.

18. Kohn, L.T., & Corrigan, J.M. (Eds.) & Donaldson, M.S. (ed.) (1999). To *Err Is Human: Building a Safer Health System.* Washington, DC: National Academy Press.

19. Lazarou, J., Pomeranz, B.H., & Corey, P.N. (1998). Incidence of adverse drug reactions in hospitalized patients. *Journal of the American Medical Association., 279*, 1200-1205.

20. Meredith, S., Feldman, P. H., Frey, D., Hall, K., Arnold, K., Brown, N. J., & Ray, W.A. (2001). Possible medication errors in home healthcare patients. *Journal of the American Geriatrics Society, 49*, 719-724.

21. Meredith, S., Feldman, P., Frey, D., Giammarco, L., Hall, K., Arnold, K., Brown, N. J., & Ray, W. A. (2002). Improving medication use in home healthcare patients: A randomized controlled trial. *JAGS, 50*,1484-1491.

22. Wilcox, S., Himmelstein, D., & Woolhandler, S. (1994). Inappropriate Drug Prescribing for the Community-Dwelling Elderly. *Journal of the American Medical Association, 272*, 292-296.

23. Zhan, C., Sangl, J., Bierman, A.S., Miller, M.R., Friedman, B., Wickizer, S.W., & Meyer, G.S. (2001). Potentially inappropriate medication use in the community-dwelling elderly. *Journal of the American Medical Association, 286*(22), 2823-2829.

24. Joint Commission of Accreditation of Healthcare Organizations. (n.d.) *2005 Home care national patient safety goals.* Retrieved August 27, 2004 from http://www.jcaho.org/accredited+organizations/home+care/npsg/05_npsg_hc.htm.

A Quality Improvement Project to Reduce Falls and Improve Medication Management

Sandy Sperling, PharmD
Katie Neal, RN, BSN, PHN
Kelly Hales, PharmD
Dale Adams, PharmD
Dennee Frey, PharmD

SUMMARY. This paper describes the implementation of a medication management model within a medical-center based home health agency. The model was integrated into the agency's quality improvement falls prevention program and was selected in part because it directly addressed two medication-related accreditation standards for home health care agencies. During a five-month period, a staff pharmacist conducted

Sandy Sperling is affiliated with the Home Care Pharmacy. Katie Neal is affiliated with Memorial Home Health Services. Kelly Hales and Dale Adams are affiliated with LBMMC- Pharmacy Administration. Dennee Frey is affiliated with Partners in Care Foundation.

Address correspondence to: Sandy Sperling, PharmD, Home Care Pharmacy, 450 Spring Street, Suite 11, Long Beach, CA 90806 (E-mail: ssperling@memorialcare.org).

This project was funded in part by the John A. Hartford Foundation, Inc., New York, New York. The Foundation awarded funding to Partners in Care Foundation to disseminate the Medication Management Model program and to provide technical assistance to leading home health providers across the country, including Memorial Home Health Care. Project results and toolkit materials can be found at *www. homemeds.org.*

[Haworth co-indexing entry note]: "A Quality Improvement Project to Reduce Falls and Improve Medication Management." Sperling, Sandy et al. Co-published simultaneously in *Home Health Care Services Quarterly* (The Haworth Press, Inc.) Vol. 24, No. 1/2, 2005, pp. 13-28; and: *Improving Medication Management in Home Care: Issues and Solutions* (ed: Dennee Frey) The Haworth Press, Inc., 2005, pp. 13-28. Single or multiple copies of this article are available for a fee from The Haworth Document Delivery Service [1-800-HAWORTH, 9:00 a.m. - 5:00 p.m. (EST). E-mail address: docdelivery@haworthpress.com].

medication reviews for 228 HHA patients who met the program's inclusion criteria. Thirty-three percent of these patients required some type of follow-up to resolve potential medication-related problems. By far, falls were the most common reason for referral, with 71 patients, or 30% of all participating patients, referred to the pharmacist due to a recent fall. From a quality improvement standpoint, the program met and even exceeded expectations in that it enabled staff to identify a serious threat to patient safety–medication-related problems, especially falls–and gave them the tools to resolve these potential problems. *[Article copies available for a fee from The Haworth Document Delivery Service: 1-800-HAWORTH. E-mail address: <docdelivery@haworthpress.com> Website: <http://www.HaworthPress. com> © 2005 by The Haworth Press, Inc. All rights reserved.]*

KEYWORDS. Medication management, medication-related problems, drug regimen review, falls prevention, continuous quality improvement, accreditation standards, and patient safety

INTRODUCTION AND PURPOSE

Older adults are at an especially high risk for medication-related problems. This is partly due to the number of diseases and changes that occur with age and in part because they take so many medications–an average of six a day, more than any other age group (Beers, 2001). One of the most serious medication-related events for the elderly is falls.

Thirty to sixty percent of community-dwelling elderly fall each year, with potentially serious consequences (Rubenstein and Josephson, 2002). Among older adults, two-thirds of accidental deaths, which rank as the fifth leading cause of death in the elderly, are due to falls (Rubenstein and Josephson, 2002). Although most falls do not result in injury, each year between 5 and 10% of community-dwelling older persons who do fall sustain a serious injury, such as a hip fracture, head injury, or laceration (Magaziner et al., 1990; Rubenstein et al., 2003). These injuries can result in long-term morbidity.

Several studies have identified risk factors that increase the likelihood of falling. Among the most important risk factors is polypharmacy. In a recent literature review, Rubenstein and Josephson (2002/3) cite a meta-analysis that found a significantly increased risk of falls from psychotropic medications and cardiac medications such as digoxin, diuretics, and antiarrhythmics. Other studies also have shown "less strong but still clinically and statistically significant relationships between use of three or more medications and risk of falls" (Rubenstein and Josephson, 2002/3). Of particular concern are other medication-related risk factors for injurious falls. A survey of Medicaid enrollees revealed that the risk of hip fracture increased two-fold for elderly adults taking psychotropic medications (Ray, Griffin, and Schaffner, 1987). An additional study indicates that elderly persons using benzodiazepines may have two to three times the risk of falls and two times the risk of hip fracture when compared to elderly nonusers. These rates are increased in women and especially in women 65 years of age or older. Moreover, women also have two to three times as many hip fractures as do men (Ensrud K.E., Blackwell T.L., Mangione C.M. et al., 2002).

Medication review is gaining recognition as a key component of effective fall prevention programs. The Medication Management Model (MMM) developed and tested by researchers at Vanderbilt University and collaborating home health agencies (HHA) provides specific guidelines for implementing these reviews, and evaluating high-risk medications for elderly home health patients (Meredith et al., 2002; Meredith et al., 2001; Brown et al., 1998).

At the same time, accreditation entities such as the Joint Commission on Accreditation of Healthcare Organizations (JCAHO) have focused standards that address a healthcare organization's level of performance in specific areas on improving patient safety as well as medication management. Starting in 2005, newly revised JCAHO standards will require home health agencies to address National Patient Safety Goals to improve the safety of using medications and to reduce the risk of patient harm resulting from falls (JCAHO, 2004).

This paper describes implementation of the MMM within a medical-center based home health agency, Memorial Home Health Care (MHHC), as part of an established Quality Improvement program. At the time it adopted the MMM, the center already was addressing the commission's patient safety goals within its performance improvement program, particularly in the area of falls.

According to JCAHO, "The standards detail important functions relating to care of individuals and the management of health care organizations. . . . Because the standards aim to improve outcomes, they place little emphasis on how to achieve these objectives" (www.jcaho.org/accredited+organizations/home+care/standards/standards.htm). In other words, healthcare agencies are free to choose their own course of action to achieve stated goals and can choose from various Performance Improvement (PI) management philosophies and theoretical models for their continuous quality improvement (CQI) process. MHHC has chosen to implement a model developed by Richard Chang, PhD, that includes five steps: *S*elect, *A*ssess, *M*easure, *I*mprove, and *E*valuate, i.e., SAMIE (Chang, 1994).

The MMM was included in this PI model (Figure 1) and expanded the HHA's ability to assess and evaluate one of its key performance improvement indicators: reducing patient falls. In the process, it also enabled the agency overall to improve medication management and minimize the occurrence of adverse events.

METHODS

Setting

MHHC provides skilled nursing, infusion therapy, hospice care, and rehabilitation (physical, occupational, and speech therapy) services to home health (HH) patients. MHHC is a division of Long Beach Memorial Medical Center (LBMMC), a 778-licensed bed facility in southern California and the second largest private hospital on the west coast. A comprehensive medical campus, LBMMC combines the resources of seven major entities: Memorial Hospital, Miller Children's Hospital, Memorial Women's Hospital, Memorial Rehabilitation Hospital, Memorial Heart Institute, Memorial Cancer Institute, and MHHC. Now in its 90th year, LBMMC is nationally recognized for excellence in health care.

Quality Improvement Program

LBMMC chose to integrate Chang's PI model into its quality improvement program for all areas and services, including home health services. In the fall of 2002, MHHC selected the Medication Management Model as its means of directly addressing two JCAHO standards for home healthcare agencies:

- Standard MM.6.10: The effects of medication(s) on patients are monitored.
- Standard MM.6.20: The organization responds appropriately to actual or potential adverse drug events and medication errors.

MHHC administrators reasoned that the MMM, apart from helping the agency better meet JCAHO standards, would blend in well with its

FIGURE 1. Medication Management Process Improvement Summary

Team Members
Pharmacist Clinical Specialist;
Vice President, Medical Services;
Executive Director, Ambulatory Pharmacy;
Executive Director of Home Health Services

SELECT

Patients 65 years of age and older frequently take multiple prescription and over-the-counter medications which are often prescribed by multiple physicians and obtained from more than one pharmacy. While hospitalized patients routinely have their medications reviewed by a pharmacist, no such review is currently required by regulatory agencies for Home Health patients. This lack of overview could potentially lead to adverse medication events.

The initial focus of the Medication Management Model at LBMMC was to have a consultant pharmacist review the medications of patients over 64 years of age on service who either had 10 or more medications on their medication profile or had had an unexplained fall within the previous 3 months. This was later expanded to include other criteria suggested by the Model, including patients with blood pressure out of range, orthostatic hypotension, bradycardia on medications that lower heart rate, or those with a recent change in mental status.

The Medication Management Model expanded MHHC's ability to address one of its ongoing performance improvement indicators, reducing patient falls.

ASSESS

Prior to implementation, HHA hospice and infusion nurses had frequent contact with other LBMMC pharmacists, since LBMMC pharmacies are contracted to provide clinical and distributive services to these patients. However, in the medical-surgical and rehabilitation populations, no such relationship between MHHC staff and pharmacists previously existed. These latter two populations receive their prescriptions from a myriad of pharmacies in the Los Angeles basin.

IMPORTANT FUNCTIONS

- Provision of Care, Treatment and Service
- Medication Management

DIMENSIONS OF PERFORMANCE

- Safety
- Appropriateness
- Continuity

MEASURE

A total of 228 patients met the inclusion criteria and were reviewed in a 5-month period from mid-January to mid-June 2003

IMPROVE

Actions for improvement include:
- Developed and expanded referral (trigger) form to be used by field staff and the supervisors to identify elderly patients who met referral criteria.
- Educate MHHC staff to the use of the referral form.
- Present pharmacist findings at MHHC staff meetings and discuss solutions to problems encountered.
- Developed direct communication linkage with patients to obtain information quickly and efficiently.
- Direct patient counseling by the pharmacist regarding the drug problem.
- Keep statistics of patients and measure outcomes/results.

EVALUATE

Direct patient contact proved to be the most effective means of problem resolution.
Increased staff awareness and better reporting increased the number of recorded falls – this represents an artificial increase.
LBMMC, with its commitment to patient care, plans to continue this program, making the pharmacist more visible to MHHC staff to facilitate communication and thus, improve ability to quickly resolve important medication issues.

performance improvement program by enhancing patient safety through medication review and oversight for at-risk patients. Of particular interest to the HHA was the model's effect on two outcome measures: patient falls and patients' ability to take oral medications. This paper focuses primarily on patient falls.

JCAHO evaluates accredited home health organizations every three years to monitor ongoing compliance with its standards. The tool used to assess performance addresses all applicable standards and Accreditation Participation Requirements (APRs), which include the commission's national patient safety goals. MHHC was due for such a review in June of 2004. As this paper will report, MHHC's decision to adopt the Medication Management Model aligned aspects of the agency's performance so closely with JCAHO expectations that it met some of the commission's 2005 patient safety goals in 2004.

Overview of Program Implementation

MHHC staff built upon the experiences of the other home health technical assistance sites to implement the Medication Management Model (see other articles in this volume). Briefly, the MMM uses guidelines established by an expert panel for resolving high-risk medication problems among home health patients. The model's intervention features a consultant pharmacist assisting the home health nurse to assess and resolve potential medication problems (Brown, 1998).

MMM participants included HHA patients age 65 and over admitted to the agency's Medicare-certified Medical-surgical, Rehabilitation, Hospice, and Infusion programs who met the referral criteria (below). Admission visits were conducted by nursing and rehabilitation therapy staff who used a referral, or trigger, form to identify patients meeting referral criteria.

Initially, the eligibility or referral criteria included elderly patients on 10 or more medications or who met at least one of the following criteria:

- Had an unexplained fall in the last three months
- Had a recent change in mental status
- Showed evidence of medication noncompliance, indication of poor medication response, or adverse effects

Later, the eligibility criteria, and consequently, the referral form (Figure 2), were expanded to include the following:

- Blood pressure greater than or equal to 160/100
- Blood pressure less than or equal to 90/50 and on a medication that can lower blood pressure
- Orthostasis greater than or equal to 20 mm Hg upon postural change
- Pulse rate less than 60 and on a medication that can reduce heart rate

This change enabled the pharmacist to determine efficacy or potential adverse effects of antihypertensive therapy and other factors relating to vasoactive and cardiac medications and conformed more closely to the original clinical protocols.

At the onset of the program, all clinical home health staff of MHHC were educated about the model and the implementation process at a monthly clinical staff meeting.

Field staff and the supervisors used the referral form to identify elderly patients who met eligibility criteria. For each at-risk patient, field or supervisory staff completed the referral form and attached copies of the patient's medication profile and "face sheet" with demographic, diagnostic, and insurance information. These materials were placed in the consultant pharmacist's mail slot, which the pharmacist checked daily.

If additional patient information was needed, the pharmacist contacted the appropriate staff member, checked the hospital computer for additional patient information including laboratory results and also frequently called the patient directly. The pharmacist monitored home health patients who were admitted to LBMMC via the hospital computer throughout their stay. With all data in hand, the pharmacist conducted a medication review. If changes to the medication regimen were indicated, the pharmacist contacted the patient's physician directly to discuss the recommendations. Field staff and the coordinators followed up with patients to ensure that any medication changes were implemented and monitored patients for potential problems.

MHHC developed a data collection tool using Excel software to track the numbers of patients reviewed as well as interventions and outcomes. This data currently is being analyzed for quality improvement purposes. MHHC staff and the consultant pharmacist also kept track of the time they spent to develop and implement the model.

RESULTS

A total of 228 patients met the inclusion criteria and were reviewed in a five-month period from mid-January to mid-June, 2003. This total in-

FIGURE 2. Medication Management Model–Triggers for Pharmacy Intervention

Instructions for use of form:

This form is to be completed for all active cases in the participating sites at the following intervals:

- SOC
- ROC
- Recertification

*In addition, the form is to be completed after learning of a fall, provided the patient remains at home and at any other time the nurse identifies a significant change in condition.

Patient Name:_____ Medical Record Number:_____ DOB:_____

Site Name & Address:_____

Physician **First** and **Last** Name:_____

Physician Phone #_____

SOC ☐   ROC ☐   Recert ☐   Recent Fall ☐   Other ☐

Please answer the following:	Yes	No
1. Does the patient take 10 or more medications per day?	☐	☐
2. Has the patient had an unexplained fall in the last 3 months?	☐	☐

Circumstances of fall: _____

_____

	Yes	No
3. Has there been a recent change in mental status?	☐	☐
4. Is there evidence of medication non-compliance or indication of poor medication response or adverse effects?	☐	☐

If yes, explain: _____

_____

5. What is the patient's blood pressure? ____/_____ (supine/sitting/standing)

6. Does the patient have orthostatic hypotension > 20mm Hg? Yes/No/Non-ambulatory

If yes, record BPs and positions:

7. What is the patient's pulse rate? _____bpm

Coments:_____

_____

Completed by: _____

Case Manager _____

Signature: _____

Pager #: _____

Team: _____

WHEN PHARMACIST INTERVENTION IS INDICATED, attach patient's medication sheet to this form and contact Rph.

cludes three patients under age 65 referred to the pharmacist, who reviewed their medications as a courtesy. Table 1 presents the breakdown of all patients by service area along with the incidence of adverse medication events recorded. Patients were counted only once, even if they went off service and then returned, or if they changed services. A drug event is recorded in more than one category if there was more than one issue, such as an inappropriate drug causing a fall.

The patients were taking an average of 13 medications each (range 2-38). Patients on fewer than 10 medications who did not meet another criterion, such as a recent fall or high blood pressure, were not referred.

Somewhat more than half (52%, n = 119) of the referred patients, were receiving home healthcare nursing through the Medical-Surgical Service. Thirty-eight percent of the patients (n = 87) were receiving rehabilitation services, i.e., physical, occupational, or speech therapy. Considerably fewer patients were receiving infusion therapy (n = 13) or hospice care (n = 8).

Falls were by far the most common reason for referral, with 71 patients, or 30% of all participating patients, referred to the pharmacist due to a recent fall. Of these 71 patients, 68% were referred from the Rehabilitation Service.

Other referrals were triggered by possible duplicative therapy (n = 23), potential drug interactions or a single drug problem (n = 11), hypertension (n = 4), orthostasis (n = 2), change in mental status (n = 2), and low heart rate (n = 1). It should be noted that patients were referred for potential cardiac problems, such as hypertension and orthostatic hypotension, only after the trigger form was revised, which may account for the lower number of referrals for these possible drug-related problems.

Falls

Further analysis of patient falls showed that at least nine (13%) were possibly or probably medication-related (Table 2). Because the initial referral form did not include sufficient information for the pharmacist to determine the circumstances surrounding a fall, she often contacted the patient directly to obtain more information. Most falls were clearly mechanical falls due to tripping, walking on uneven surfaces, and even falling while dancing. Less frequent occurrences were falls upon transfer due to lower extremity weakness and falls from stroke.

When a fall was determined to be possibly medication-related, the pharmacist took action to re-evaluate the drug implicated. Some drugs

TABLE 1. Patient Referrals by Clinical Area

Area	Number of Patients	Age Range			Average Number of Medications[1]	Duplicate Therapy[2]	Drug Event[3]	Criteria for Pharmacist Review					
		Average Age	Youngest	Oldest				Falls[4]	Hypertension[5]	Hypotension[6]	Orthostasis[7]	Low Heart Rate[8]	Change in Mental Status[9]
Medical/Surgical	117	79	60	98	13	14	6	22	2	0	0	0	2
Physical Therapy	87	79	52	96	10	4	5	48	2	0	2	0	0
Hospice	8	86	76	107	13	2	0	1	0	0	0	0	0
Infusion	13	75	66	100	15	3	0	0	0	0	0	0	0
Multiple Disciplines	3	82	74	87	15	0	0	0	0	0	0	1	0
Averages		80	52	107	13								
Totals (n)	228					23	11	71	4	0	2	1	2
Percentage (%)	100					11	5	31	2	0	0.9	0.4	0.9

Notes:
1. Average number of medications in patients reviewed. Being on 10 or more medications was one referral criterion. Patients on fewer medications who met another criterion are included.
2. Duplication of therapy based on medication profile.
3. Drug interaction or single drug problem.
4. A fall could be the precipitating event for home health care or it could occur after home health care is started for another reason.
5. Blood pressure greater than or equal to 160/100. The Tool Kit suggested using 180/110, but it was reasonable to follow-up with anything that appeared high in view of new AHA recommendations.
6. Blood pressure less than or equal to 90/50 on a medication that can lower blood pressure.
7. Orthostasis greater than or equal to 20 mm Hg upon postural change.
8. Pulse less than 60 on a medication that can reduce heart rate.
9. Recent change in mental status.

TABLE 2. Possible Medication-Related Falls (n = 9)

• Patient with orthostatic hypotension erroneously received a prescription for promethazine instead of ProAmatine
• Patient lost balance due to imipramine use
• Patient did not eat after taking glipizide and fell from apparent hypoglycemia
• Patient was taking two benzodiazepines and a narcotic
• Patient says prednisone caused dizziness and a fall
• Patient was taking Klonopin 1.5 mg daily and fell in the shower
• Ativan was administered for two doses before a fall
• Overdiuresis caused hyponatremia, hypokalemia, and hypovolemia, leading to a fall
• Patient on terazosin turned quickly and fell

were discontinued or the dosage reduced by the attending physician based on the pharmacist's recommendation.

Implementation Process

In five months of operation, the pharmacist averaged approximately four hours per week to set up the medication management system; review medications for 228 patients; revise referral criteria; contact patients, staff and physicians; and attend a minimal number of staff meetings.

Approximately six hours were needed at the outset to develop the referral system with managers and staff (4 hours) and create, test and modify the Excel database (2 hours). Time requirements for ongoing operations were fairly minimal for field staff: approximately 10 minutes for each referred patient. The pharmacist spent approximately 10 minutes per patient to process data, including reviewing patient information and entering it into the Excel database. The pharmacist spent another 10 minutes per targeted patient on phone calls to nurses, rehab therapists, physicians, and patients to gather the additional information needed for a comprehensive medication review. She spent additional time monitoring patients via the hospital's computer and attending administrative meetings.

DISCUSSION

Patient Distribution

As expected, the vast majority of the 228 referred patients came from the Medical-Surgical (52%) and Rehabilitation (38%) Services. Prior to the start of this program, healthcare providers with these services had only infrequent contact with pharmacists, unlike field staff with the Hospice and Infusion Services, who interact regularly with pharmacists supporting those programs.

Most medical-surgical patients over 65 years of age met the criterion of taking ten or more medications. This population had never previously had medication profiles systematically reviewed. Thirty-five patients (29%) in this group required follow-up.

As expected, the greatest number of falls was reported in patients on the Rehabilitation Service. In some cases the fall was the precipitating event for home health care (such as a fall that caused a hip fracture). In others, it occurred after the start of care. Increased staff awareness and better reporting increased the number of recorded falls during this period.

Thirty-four patients (39%) on the Rehabilitation Service required follow-up, some with medication issues unrelated to falls. MHHC rehabilitation patients are not admitted by nurses, but by physical, occupational, and speech therapists, who generally do not have an extensive background in drug therapy issues. Given this, it is perhaps not surprising that the pharmacist discovered a significant number of medication-related problems among these patients.

Less than 10% of the referred patients were on hospice or receiving infusion therapy. Most MHHC infusion patients were under age 65 and thus ineligible for medication review under this program. Most MHHC hospice patients met the age criterion but did not screen in for review because they were taking fewer than 10 medications as their care shifted from treatment to palliation. However, these patients received close monitoring by Hospice/Infusion pharmacists.

Overall, 67% (n = 154) of the referred patients did not require further follow-up by the pharmacist. Most problems could be resolved through patient counseling without having to contact the physician directly to change orders. In certain cases, if a patient with a non-urgent medication issue had a pending appointment with the physician, he or she was instructed to follow up with a specific question to the doctor at that time.

Quality Improvement

From a quality improvement standpoint, the MMM met and even exceeded expectations in that it enabled staff to identify a serious threat to patient safety–that is, medication-related problems, especially falls–and gave them the tools to resolve these potential problems. Administrators report that field staff got into a "safety mode" so that by the time the JCAHO accreditation survey occurred, the activity was ongoing for them.

Details of each step of the improvement process are summarized in Figure 1. In evaluating the findings, it was noted that increased staff awareness and better reporting increased the number of recorded falls during this period, possibly representing an artificial increase. Thus a change in data collection was initiated to separate the "falls" information into four categories: falls occurring prior to admission or after admission to Home Health, and for each of these, whether or not the fall was possibly or probably medication-related.

During its JCAHO accreditation visit in June 2004, MHHC received positive feedback from the survey team for effectively addressing both medication management and patient safety goals by implementing the model. Additionally, MHHC had anticipated the Joint Commission's 2005 National Patient Safety Goals, published almost a year after the agency adopted the Medication Management Model. Among them is the following goal, which links falls and medication management:

- Reduce the risk of patient harm resulting from falls: Assess and periodically reassess each patient's risk for falling, including the potential risk associated with the patient's medication regimen, and take action to address any identified risks. (JCAHO, 2004)

At the time of its JCAHO review, MHHC was already taking such action and had been working to reduce patient fall risk for months.

Though staff initially had to work through a trial-and-error stage to establish effective communication channels and referral protocols for the new medication review program, ultimately the model proved feasible to implement and maintain. Case studies presented by the pharmacist helped the home health staff, especially medical-surgical nurses and rehab therapists, who previously had only limited experience working with pharmacists, to see a tangible connection between their new screening and referral responsibilities under the program and resultant positive outcomes for their patients. The SAMIE evaluation recommended increasing pharmacist visibility to MHHC staff to facilitate communication and thus, to improve the team's ability to effectively resolve important medication issues.

One unexpected outcome of the program was the positive interaction between the pharmacist and home health patients. Because of challenges in reaching field staff for additional information needed for the medication reviews, the pharmacist directly contacted many of the patients by telephone. Though the majority of patients were over age 80, most were able to converse cogently about their medication use and its effects and, among those who had had a recent fall, most were able to recount the circumstances of the fall. If the patient was unable to communicate, the spouse or caregiver often was able to provide this information. Direct contact with patients enabled the pharmacist to obtain needed information quickly and efficiently, ask additional questions that may not have been anticipated had field staff followed-up, and resolve numerous concerns through a single phone call. Overall these were felt to be positive communications; nearly every patient contacted appreciated the call and the opportunity to discuss their medications with a qualified professional. The improvement team concluded that direct patient contact proved to be the most effective means of problem resolution.

Implementation Barriers

The initial referral form did not provide the pharmacist with sufficient information to evaluate a patient's medication regimen. Modifications to the form corrected this problem by including additional clinical information such as blood pressure and details about falls.

Some clinical staff resisted the additional paperwork at the onset of the program. As a result, referral forms sometimes were incomplete, hampering the pharmacist's ability to complete medication reviews. At the same time, the pharmacist perhaps was not visible enough to MHHC staff, in part because she viewed the resolution of medication-related problems as the program's endpoint. These teamwork issues were largely resolved through case presentations by the pharmacist, which provided valuable feedback on outcomes to nurses and therapists, thereby completing the circle of communication, a hallmark characteristic of continuous quality improvement programs.

Also at the start of the program, the pharmacist was inundated with as many as 80 referrals at one time as MHHC sought to screen all eligible patients. This led to a time delay (about 3-7 days) between admission to the agency and a review of the patient's medications. Several patients from this initial group of referrals were off service by the time follow-up was attempted.

Limitations

Inclusion criteria for the Medication Management Model were fairly rigorous to adhere to the original model and to focus the pharmacist's time. Consequently, there likely were other patients who could have benefited from the program. It was beyond the scope of this phase of the project, however, to attempt to optimize admission screening criteria further.

CONCLUSION

This field test demonstrated the value of the Medication Management Model as a program that can help expand a HHA's ability to address one of its ongoing performance improvement indicators, reducing patient falls. It addresses important functions in providing care and treatment across home health services, particularly for older medical-surgical and rehabilitation patients at risk for possible medication-related problems. An agency can meet and even anticipate challenging accreditation standards while enhancing patient safety. A staff or consultant pharmacist with expertise in evaluating drug therapies is essential to the program. Based on the positive results of the project, MHHC is maintaining the Medication Management intervention for its patients, and fall prevention continues to be a primary goal of its quality improvement program.

REFERENCES

Beers M. (2001). Age-related changes as a risk factor for medication-related problems. *Generations, 4*, 22-27.

Brown N., Griffin M., Ray W., Meredith S., Beers M., Marren J., Robles M., Stergachis A., Wood A., and Avorn J. (1998). A model for improving medication use in home health care patients. *Journal of the American Pharmaceutical Association, 38*, 696-702.

Chang R. (1994). *Continuous process improvement (Quality improvement series).* Richard Chang Associates, Inc.

Ensrud K., Blackwell T., Mangione C., Bowman P., Whooley M., Bauer D., Schwartz A., Hanlon J., and Nevitt M. (2002). Central nervous system-active medications and risk for falls in older women. *Journal of the American Geriatrics Society, 50,* 1629-1637.

2005 Home care national patient safety goals. Retrieved August 27, 2004 from Joint Commission on Accreditation of Healthcare Organizations Web Site: http://www.jcaho.org/accredited+organizations/home+care/npsg/05_npsg_hc.htm.

Magaziner J., Simonsick E.M., Kashner T.M., Hebel J.R., and Kenzora J.E. (1990). Predictors of functional recovery one year following hospital discharge for hip fracture: A prospective study. *Journal of Gerontology: Medical Sciences, 45,* M101.

Meredith S., Feldman P.H., Frey D., Hall K., Arnold K., Brown N.J., and Ray W.A. (2001). Possible medication errors in home healthcare patients. *Journal of the American Geriatrics Society, 49,* 719-724.

Meredith S., Feldman P., Frey D., Giammarco L., Hall K., Arnold K., Brown N.J., and Ray W.A. (2002). Improving medication use in newly admitted home healthcare patients: A randomized controlled trial. *Journal of the American Geriatrics Society, 50,* 1484-1491.

Ray W.A., Griffin M.R., and Schaffner W. (1987). Psychotropic drug use and the risk of hip fracture. *New England Journal of Medicine, 316,* 363-369.

Rubenstein L.Z. and Josephson K.R. (2002/03). Risk factors for falls: A central role in prevention. *Generations, 26,* 15-21.

Rubenstein L.Z. and Josephson K.R. (2002). The epidemiology of falls and syncope. *Clinics in Geriatric Medicine, 18,* 141-158.

Rubenstein L.Z., Castle S.C., Diener D.D., Hooker S.P., Jones C.J., and Vasquez L. (2003). Best practice interventions for fall prevention. Prepared for *A California Blueprint for Fall Prevention Conference,* sponsored by the Archstone Foundation.

Integration
of a Medication Management Model into Outcome-Based Quality Improvement: A Pilot Program in a Rural Proprietary Home Healthcare Agency

Wayne L. Atkinson, RPh CGP
Dennee Frey, PharmD

Wayne L. Atkinson is Clinical Pharmacist Consultant, Home Care Plus, Lewisburg, WV. Dennee Frey is affiliated with the Partners in Care Foundation.

Address correspondence to: Wayne L. Atkinson, RPh, CGP, Clinical Pharmacist Consultant, Home Care Plus, HC 81 Box 288, Lewisburg, WV 24901 (E-mail: wla2@charter.net).

Special acknowledgment is extended to the management and staff of Home Care Plus, in particular, the ongoing support of Pam Wigglesworth, RN, Owner and CEO, and Lois Hayslett, RN, Quality Manager for Home Care Plus, who ensured the successful implementation of this project. Acknowledgement is also extended to management of Allegheny Software Publishers, Inc., St. Marys, PA. Their expertise and support ensured the successful development and implementation of the computerized patient risk screens utilized in this project.

This project was funded in part by the John A. Hartford Foundation, Inc., New York, New York. The Foundation awarded funding to Partners in Care Foundation to disseminate the Medication Management Model program and to provide technical assistance to leading home health providers across the country, including Home Care Plus. Project results and toolkit materials can be found at *www.homemeds.org*.

[Haworth co-indexing entry note]: "Integration of a Medication Management Model into Outcome-Based Quality Improvement: A Pilot Program in a Rural Proprietary Home Healthcare Agency." Atkinson, Wayne L., and Dennee Frey. Co-published simultaneously in *Home Health Care Services Quarterly* (The Haworth Press, Inc.) Vol. 24, No. 1/2, 2005, pp. 29-45; and: *Improving Medication Management in Home Care: Issues and Solutions* (ed: Dennee Frey) The Haworth Press, Inc., 2005, pp. 29-45. Single or multiple copies of this article are available for a fee from The Haworth Document Delivery Service [1-800-HAWORTH, 9:00 a.m. - 5:00 p.m. (EST). E-mail address: docdelivery@haworthpress.com].

SUMMARY. This article describes a rural proprietary home health agency's successful initiative to adapt a previously tested medication management model and integrate it into existing processes of care. The rationale to improve medication management in response to current national fiscal, clinical and external quality measures and evolution of this process in the agency is detailed. The agency refined the model's screening procedures, incorporating them into the mandated OASIS assessment and then computerizing the medication risk analysis, in keeping with the original intent of the model. In a four-month pilot test of the computerized risk assessment procedure 1006 OASIS assessments were screened; risk factors for medication-related problems in 201 (19.9%) resulted in pharmacist review. Of these, 30 (17%) were ruled out as potential medication errors, 143 (82.6%) were found with potential MRP and 58 (33.5%) had evidence of problems warranting follow-up. With this computer-assisted process, the agency created a more comprehensive assessment that was in line with the new regulatory emphasis on patient outcomes. Consultant pharmacist services also transitioned from drug regimen review to more comprehensive medication therapy management. By enhancing efficiencies in its medication management program, an agency not only stands to improve quality of care, but also to maximize resources, making the intervention affordable to implement and decreasing burden on staff. *[Article copies available for a fee from The Haworth Document Delivery Service: 1-800-HAWORTH. E-mail address: <docdelivery@haworthpress.com> Website: <http://www.HaworthPress.com>*

KEYWORDS. OASIS assessment, medication therapy management, OBQI, home health care, pharmacist interventions, model of care

INTRODUCTION

Recent financial, regulatory, and marketing changes in the home health industry provide compelling reasons for agencies to improve their medication management practices. These far-reaching changes include declining reimbursement under a Prospective Payment System (PPS), required utilization of a standardized patient assessment focused on outcome measures, and a national quality improvement initiative that features publicly available quality reports for virtually every home health agency (HHA). In addition, the recently enacted Medicare Modernization Act of 2003 (www.cms.hhs.gov/medicareform/) provides for

Medicare beneficiaries to receive medication therapy management services as part of an outpatient pharmacy benefit that begins in 2006. An overview of each of these changes follows.

THE PROSPECTIVE PAYMENT SYSTEM

Under the PPS, HHAs are paid a fixed amount for each episode of care regardless of the patient's length of stay or number of home visits. In this way the system provides a financial incentive for providers to limit stays and reduce the number of home health visits. The advent of PPS in 2000 caused some HHAs to close for financial reasons. Many of the agencies that survived the payment reform renewed their focus on clinical issues, and in particular, on innovative strategies for effectively managing patient care within the current reimbursement system. In this respect, improved medication management can help HHAs control for extended-stay risk by promptly resolving medication problems and promoting optimal health.

Required Assessments and Outcome Reports

Federal home health regulations introduced along with the PPS also have provided an incentive to improve medication management. These regulations require HHAs to regularly monitor medications as part of a standardized patient assessment. The federal Centers for Medicare and Medicaid Services (CMS) analyzes data from this assessment, called the Outcomes and Assessment Information Set or OASIS, and reports it back to agencies as clinical outcomes measures.

In a related change, CMS in 2001 launched a home health care adverse event reporting system based on Outcome-Based Quality Improvement (OBQI) reports. Under mandate from CMS, state departments of health create such reports for all HHAs that provide skilled services to Medicare and Medicaid patients. CMS has chosen thirteen adverse or "untoward" events as "red flags" that indicate serious quality-of-care problems. Among these are emergent care for improper medication administration or side effects, and declines in patient function due to noncompliance with a recommended medication regimen.

The value of using patient outcome reports to improve the quality of home health care has been reported by Shaughnessy et al. (2002), who found that such reports "had a pervasive effect on outcome improvements for home health patients." Compared to a control group of HHAs, agencies that received patient outcome reports and used them to target their improvement efforts showed a significantly higher rate of decline in hospitalizations over two years as well as improvements in outcome measures of health status. In an editorial response (2002), Dr. Peter Boling of the Virginia Commonwealth University called the Shaughnessy study "a landmark event in home care research," one that "reflects the leading edge of a sea change in Medicare home health services." Regulatory attention to poor clinical outcomes along with feedback from the OBQI reports has prompted some HHAs to adopt medication management projects that aim to reduce the number of medication-related adverse events.

Home Health Quality Measures

Another impetus for changing medication management practices is that CMS now publishes "Home Health Quality Measures" that list 11 quality measures for each of the nation's Medicare-certified HHAs (Appendix). Of these measures, five are especially sensitive to medication selection and management: improvement in toileting, improved medication management, reduced frequency of confusion, improved pain management, and prevention of acute hospitalization and emergency room use. Available online and in print to help consumers make informed choices about home health care, these report cards have the potential to invigorate prevention management practices, including medication management, within HHAs (see Authors' Note).

Medication Management Therapy Services

Medicare's new prescription drug benefit for seniors also is expected to reshape home health medication management, as it offers a potential new reimbursement opportunity. Starting in 2006, prescription drug plans that offer the new, expanded drug benefit will be required to have a medication therapy management program to ensure the appropriate use of prescription drugs to improve outcomes and reduce adverse drug interactions (CMS, 2004). Though the plans will have some flexibility, in general, these programs will pay pharmacists to spend time counseling patients, and will be directed at patients who:

- have multiple chronic conditions (such as asthma, diabetes, hypertension, high cholesterol and congestive heart failure);
- are taking multiple medications; and
- are likely to have high drug expenses.

CMS (2004) notes that, "like the rest of the drug benefit, medication therapy management will be a new service for Medicare. Currently, a few state Medicaid programs reimburse pharmacists for providing these 'cognitive services.'"

Taken together, these industry-wide changes have created and will continue to create new pressures for HHAs to do more–manage service use, achieve good clinical outcomes, minimize or avoid adverse events–with less. While the changes pose challenges to HHAs, they also present an opportunity for innovation.

In our computer age, one way to innovate and maximize resources is to automate tasks. This article describes a successful initiative to implement a pharmacist-centered medication management program into the existing care practices at Home Care Plus (HCP), one of four agencies who received technical assistance to adapt the previously studied Medication Management Model (MMM). In the process, it also describes how Home Care Plus integrated the new program–and reduced the work burden on field staff–by incorporating the medication screening, or patient assessment, into the OASIS assessment and computerizing the prescreening of patients at high-risk for medication related problems.

METHODS

Agency Profile

Home Care Plus is a locally owned and managed proprietary, certified HHA serving Lewisburg, West Virginia and five surrounding counties. For nearly 20 years the agency has been providing an array of skilled and supportive home health services to over 1000 patients annually in their homes, including assisted living and nursing facilities. Services include nursing care, physical therapy, occupational therapy, speech pathology services, medical social services, and home health aid services.

The Medication Management Program

Home Care Plus was one of four HHAs that agreed to field test the Medication Management Model (described elsewhere in this volume) as a means of improving medication use among elderly patients and preventing adverse drug events (ADE). Initially, the agency identified high-risk patients and initiated pharmacist consultations using a Geriatric Medication Assessment Protocol (GMAP) (Figure 1) adapted from protocols from previous study of the model (Brown et al., 1998; Meredith et al., 2001). The GMAP targeted patients aged 65 or older who presented with one or more of four risk factors for ADEs: therapeutic duplication, cardiovascular complications, a recent fall, and recent onset of confusion. Using this protocol or screening tool, field nurses manually screened new, readmitted, and recertified patients age 65 or older for risk factors for potential ADEs. If a patient presented with one or more of the factors, the field nurse or the supervising Quality Manager submitted a request for a pharmacist consultation.

For this program, Home Care Plus contracted with a local consultant pharmacist who is also a certified geriatric pharmacist, experienced in providing geriatric pharmaceutical care in long-term and community care settings. The pharmacist was paid a flat annual fee for consultation services up to a specified number of hours.

For each consultation request, the pharmacist conducted a drug regimen review based on the model's criteria, assessing the patient for potential inappropriate medications, ADEs, and negative health outcomes potentially related to medication use. The pharmacist's written findings, assessment, recommendations, and suggested patient monitoring were forwarded to agency staff and the patient's attending physician.

Initial Results

Between January and June 1, 2003, field nurses at HCP screened 234 patients at least once for potential medication-related problems. Twenty-two percent required subsequent intervention by the consultant pharmacist. Of these, 29 (12.3%) received a written consultation to field staff and/or the physician. Analysis of GMAP outcome data showed an overall implementation rate of 36% for the pharmacist's medication recommendations (28.5% acceptance rate from physicians and 38.4% from staff).

Program Limitations

Although the GMAP successfully introduced effective clinical pharmacist assessment and intervention into existing agency care processes, the program's limitations quickly became apparent. Its most significant drawback was that it required a manual patient assessment that was not integrated with the agency's established OASIS assessment process. Given current cost constraints and mandated OASIS assessments, it is

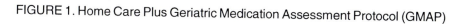

FIGURE 1. Home Care Plus Geriatric Medication Assessment Protocol (GMAP)

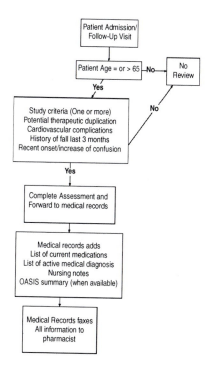

not cost-effective for agencies to conduct secondary assessments separate from the OASIS. Another drawback was that the program failed to incorporate into the risk assessment process clinically important patient and medical history information–information that is routinely collected during OASIS assessments.

In light of these limitations, and given the growing emphasis on consumer and regulatory quality outcome measures, HCP asked its software vendor to develop an automated, computer-generated medication risk assessment that would be based on a patient's OASIS assessment data and current medication regimen. Such a risk assessment process would enable the agency to meet new demands to "do more with less." Computerized medication risk assessments could be conducted more efficiently and would be more comprehensive for being based on a broader array of patient information. At the same time they would not burden field nurses with additional new tasks.

Computerized Medication Risk Assessments

The first step toward developing a computerized risk assessment program was to identify relevant data elements within the OASIS assessment reflective of the agency care process, appropriate medication selection and management, and current regulatory and consumer quality initiatives. Discussions among agency managers and staff, the clinical pharmacist, the software vendor, and the MMM project director resulted in the identification of several data elements for the preliminary patient medication risk assessment (Table 1). This initial work was based in part on a computerized risk assessment algorithm developed by researchers at Vanderbilt University for the RCT (Meredith, 2002) and available on the web at <www.homemeds.org>.

Each data element reflects a specific risk factor for medication-related problems. Among these is a primary diagnosis of congestive heart failure (CHF), which the agency added to its initial list of model-based medication risk factors because it had previously identified improvement of dyspnea for patients with CHF as a quality outcome goal.

The software vendor then created a program that would query the agency's patient database for these data elements, or risk factors, and in doing so, identify patients at high risk for medication-related problems. More specifically, the software program identifies patients who screen in with potential medication-related problems as defined by specific codes in *International Classification of Diseases, 9th Revision* (better known as ICD-9) and OASIS/Comprehensive Assessment database MO points. For example, patients at risk for falls can be identified by such ICD codes as gait disturbances (781.2), fractures (829.0), syncope (458.2), and dizziness (780.4). Patients with confusion can be identified through such MO points as MO 550 and severity rating MO 230 2-4.

Computerized Assessment Field Test

Upon successfully installing the database query for generating medication risk assessments, the agency began a four-week field test. By Tuesday of each week, medical records personnel would enter into the agency's patient database all of the previous week's OASIS assessments. Each Wednesday morning, the same staff would generate a medication risk assessment report based on the newly entered OASIS data. This report would identify patients with recent OASIS assessments who were at high risk for medication-related problems.

TABLE 1. Computerized Patient Outcome and Drug Risk Screen Criteria

Criteria Comprehensive Nursing Assessment Start of Care/Resumption of Care	Threshold for Inclusion
History of fall	≥ 2 falls during last 3 months
Pulse rate	≤ 55
Systolic blood pressure	≥ 180 or ≤ 100
Diastolic blood pressure	≥100
Orthostatic hypotension	Positive finding
Frequency of pain	Level 3–All the time
Elimination status	Urinary incontinent frequency level 3– four to six times weekly
Cognitive function	All recorded results
Mood	Frequency of anxious or depressive feelings–all recorded findings
Behavioral	Reported or observed–all recorded findings
Medical history	Primary diagnosis of Congestive Heart Failure
Potential Therapeutic Medication Duplication Report	Identification of potential therapeutic duplication. Risk screen criteria are based on therapeutic indications as well as side effect profile.

RESULTS

Each of the four weekly reports was generated without difficulty. Overall, the agency completed 161 OASIS assessments during the field test. Of this total, 86 (53.4%) were start-of-care or resumption-of-care assessments and 75 (46.6%) were re-certification-of-care assessments.

The computerized risk assessment identified a total of 44 patients (27.3%) with the following risk criteria (one patient could present with more than one criterion):

- 17 patients with a primary diagnosis of CHF (10.5%)
- 15 patients with a fall history (9.3%)
- 8 patients with presence of chronic pain (4.9%)
- 8 patients with potential cardiovascular complications (4.9%)

No patients with urinary incontinence occurring 4 to 6 times weekly were identified during the field test. With adjustments for patients identified with more than one medication risk factor, we found that 44 patients, or 27.3% of those with OASIS assessments during this four-week period, were at risk for potential medication-related problems.

Integrating Risk Assessment Agencywide

On the strength of this field test, the agency decided to incorporate the computerized medication risk assessment procedure into its routine care practices. Medical Records (MR) staff or the consultant pharmacist currently generate weekly risk assessment reports that are used by the consultant for the identification of potential medication-related problems. In addition, the software has recently been modified so that it automatically screens the agency's drug database for patients with potential therapeutic duplication. MR staff has classified each of the medications listed in the drug database into one of 41 categories; patients taking more than one medication within a selected category are identified in the weekly medication risk assessment report. Outcome data collection also has been modified to provide a future analysis of the overall impact upon utilization and intervention rates of this additional risk assessment tool.

A subsequent analysis of the medication therapy management services for the period August 1, 2003 through December 31, 2003 indicates that a total of 1006 patients with recent OASIS assessments were automatically screened (Table 2). In these screenings, 382 risk factors for medication-related problems were identified among 201 patients (19.9% of all patients with OASIS assessments; patients can present with more than one criterion). The consultant pharmacist reviewed medications for all 201 patients: reviews for 173 patients were completed within the study period; 17 patients were discharged prior to the completion of the review process; and 11 patient reviews were pending completion at the end of the study period.

Of the 173 patients with competed reviews, there was evidence of a potential problem in 143 (82.6%). The consultant pharmacist assessed 30 (17.3%) to be negative for any significant medication-related problems. After further review, including discussions with staff and/or patients and their caregivers, the pharmacist determined that 85 patients (49.1%) had several patient-medication-related characteristics that eliminated further interventions in this subgroup. These included

- patients identified as receiving palliative/terminal care
- falls assessed to be related only to environmental factors

TABLE 2. Medication Therapy Management Services Agency OASIS Assessments from August-December, 2003

No.	
OASIS assessments completed 2003 (all types)	1285
OASIS assessments "Discharged from Agency"	279
OASIS assessments (all types other than "Discharged from Agency")	1006
OASIS assessments identifying heart failure (excluding "Discharged from Agency")	115
OASIS assessments identifying falls within last 3 months (excluding "Discharged from Agency")	122
OASIS assessments identifying cardiovascular criteria (excluding "Discharged from Agency")[1]	71
OASIS assessments identifying persistent pain (excluding "Discharged from Agency")	74

1Hypertension (SBP > 180; DBP > 110) Hypotension (SBP < 100) Bradycardia (BPM < 55); Orthostatic hypotension

- duplicate therapy identified as appropriate, such as combination antihypertensive therapy
- identification of additional diagnosis and/or co-morbidity altering preliminary assessment, and
- patient desired no further interventions

The remaining 58 patients (33.5%) were identified as having a medication-related problem requiring additional intervention and management (Table 3).

DISCUSSION

The intent of technical assistance was to assist the agency in adapting the MMM into everyday field practice. On-site consultation by Partners MMM Project Director helped the agency to identify the focus of their medication improvement activity and to assess capacity to program a computerized screening tool. Participation gave the HHA an opportunity to hire a consultant pharmacist for the pharmacist-centered intervention. The agency successfully adopted the model, integrated it agency-wide with minimal cost and continues to sustain the pharmacist intervention.

TABLE 3. Medication Therapy Management Interventions for the Period August-December 2003

Patient/caregiver interventions involving direct phone contact.	58
Agency staff contact involving direct phone contact and fax communications	7
Physician contact via fax communication	9

As discussed, the agency first tested the GMAP manual risk assessment, based on a paper trigger-tool developed by another one of the technical assistance sites (FN: see www.homemeds.org). This proved to be a useful process to introduce the MMM to the agency and had particular value as a staff training tool. However, the agency wished to avoid any additional paperwork burden on staff encumbered by myriad mandated forms, an issue considered by the original investigation team in developing this model (Brown et al., 1998).

The decision to develop a computerized drug data base screening was an important step in conforming with the original model and study where the investigators assumed that potential problems are identified through routine screening of the data collected at admission (Brown et al., 1998). The complex computerized program developed by the Vanderbilt team and used for the RTC could not be used in adaptation. However, an algorithm developed by a member of the original investigation team for the project toolkit successfully guided the development of the current computer program with the agency's software vendor.

HCP decided to expand its initial list of model-based risk factors in consideration of statewide quality outcome goals and the Home Health Quality Measures. The computerized screening thus included a primary diagnosis of CHF and an indication of dyspnea, and an indication of sub-optimal pain management. Each of these conformed to the model researchers' definition of a medication problem as a pattern of medication use (or under use) and patient signs or symptoms that indicated potential sub-optimal treatment warranting reassessment of the patient (Meredith et al., 2002).

The manual or GMAP screening identified 22% of patients had a potential medication-related problem, the initial integrated computerized screening field test identified 27% of patients. In the more comprehensive four month pilot, almost 20% had negative health outcomes apparently related to medications use or under use. These findings are consistent with the model prevalence study where a possible medication error was identified for 19% of patients according to the Home Health Criteria, 17% using the Beers criteria, and 30% considering both (Meredith et al., 2001). (The findings also can be compared to another recent report that inappropriate medication usage by community-dwelling elders is between 12% and 40% (Zhan, Sangl, & Bierman, 2001)).

The pilot phase also provided valuable data about the ratio of assessments screened and yield for pharmacist review. These results suggest that an HHA that adopted this type of computer-assisted medication management program could expect that, for every 1000 OASIS assessments completed, approximately 200 consultant pharmacist reviews would be generated. In this pilot approximately 20% of the patients screened in with potential problems needing review, and approximately 6% of total (n = 58) needed comprehensive medication management interventions to resolve actual problems. This process can optimize the use of consultant services while minimizing the cost to an agency by focusing on those at highest risk.

Including OASIS patient health and functional outcomes into the computerized risk assessment differs from the usual computerized drug utilization review–widely used but criticized for lack of evidence of benefit, for producing clinically relevant alerts and for failure to consider under-use of effective medications (Meredith & Ray, 1999)–in that it has been designed to screen for problems specific to this vulnerable population.

Additionally, this approach allowed the overall clinical pharmacy service to transition from the model's DUR coordinator role (similar to the long-term therapy pharmacy drug regimen review or DRR process) toward a more comprehensive medication therapy management intervention. The model's RCT utilized experienced clinical pharmacists as DUR coordinators to improve medication management and patient outcomes through a structured intervention with home care staff and the patient's physician. The coordinator's role was to educate the HH nurse about medications and the guidelines for problem resolution, to provide clinical consultation for difficult cases and to give the nurse sufficient confidence to be able to discuss the problem with the MD (Meredith & Ray, 1999).

Medication therapy management expands the identification of drug-related problems beyond the traditional focus on "unnecessary drugs" to include such medication-related problems as untreated or under treatment of chronic conditions, improper drug selection, adverse drug reactions, and failure to receive medication. Goals of such a service are congruent with the evidence-based MMM model: to reduce polypharmacy or duplicate medications; to alert the prescriber when an individual has an apparent untreated condition that warrants drug therapy; and to assist the prescriber in monitoring whether desired therapeutic outcomes occur.

HCP's pharmacist services expanded into the realm of medication therapy management by providing comprehensive review of the patient's drug regimen, often by directly contacting the patient; evaluation of outcomes of drug therapy; and collaboration with healthcare providers such as the home health staff and prescribers to provide feedback on drug therapy.

The transition to a patient-centered medication therapy management service allowed the HCP's clinical pharmacy service to focus on the health outcomes that affect patients' functional status and quality of life, and that are potentially reversible or ameliorated through improved drug selection and management. It is an approach that is significant to this agency's outcome-based quality improvement focus and may position the agency for reimbursement for medication management services for high risk patients under the Medicare Drug Act in 2006.

It was beyond the scope of this pilot project to measure the outcomes of the pharmacist intervention. The Vanderbilt RCT demonstrated positive results with the pharmacist intervention: medication use improved for 50% of intervention patients and 38% of controls; the intervention effect was greatest for therapeutic duplication, 71% vs. 24% and cardiovascular medication use, 55% vs. 18% (Meredith et al., 2002). Other recent research has demonstrated the effectiveness of pharmacist-conducted medication management programs in home health (Triller, Clause, & Bricelan, 2000). Documented benefits include identification of potential drug-related problems such as ADEs, inappropriate dosing, poor compliance, inappropriate or inadequate monitoring, and unnecessary or incorrect drug therapy. This approach also was proven effective in eliminating duplicate therapy. Further studies of the outcomes of such evidence-based, practical interventions are needed to determine the benefits on patient function and possible positive impacts on cost, e.g., by decreasing drug costs from duplicative drugs.

CONCLUSION

A pilot project in a rural proprietary HHA demonstrated that the Medication Management Model can be successfully implemented and integrated with other assessment processes such as OASIS. Starting with a manual medication risk assessment process, the agency developed, tested, and implemented an automated weekly query of its OASIS and medication databases as a means of effectively and efficiently identifying high-risk patients with negative health outcomes that are potentially reversible with improved medication management and clinical pharmacist services. Results were consistent with the prevalence study of the evidence-based model.

The comprehensive assessment process in line with the new regulatory emphasis on patient outcomes has potential significance for quality improvement programs in other agencies. The model's clinical pharmacist intervention may qualify for reimbursement for medication therapy management services under the new Medicare Drug Act effective in 2006.

AUTHORS' NOTE

Consumers can now access the measures at two websites: Home Health Compare at *<http://www.medicare.gov/HHCompare/Home.asp?version=alternate&browser=IE%7C6%7CWin98&language=English&defaultstatus=0&pagelist=Home>*, and Home Health Quality Initiative Overview March 21, 2003 at *<http://www.cms.hhs.gov/quality/hhqi/HHQIOverview.pdf>*.

The Vanderbilt University study and results can be found at *http://www.homemeds.org* in the Visiting Nurse Services NY profile.

REFERENCES

Boling, P. (2002). Home care enhances important outcomes using OASIS and structured quality improvement. *Journal of the American Geriatrics Society, 50*, 1456-1457.

Brown, N.J., Griffin, M.R., Ray, W.A., Meredith, S., Beers, M.H., Marren, J., Robles, M., Stergachis, A., Wood, A.J.J., and Avorn, J. (1998). A model for improving medication use in home health care patients. *Journal of the American Pharmacists Association, 38*, 696-702.

Centers for Medicare and Medicaid Services. Quality improvement. Available at: http://www.cms.hhs.gov/medicarereform/issuepapers/title1and2/files/issue_paper_13_-_quality_improvements.pdf. Accessed on September 1, 2004.

Meredith, S., Feldman, P.H., Frey, D., Hall, K., Arnold, K., Brown, N.J., and Ray, W.A. (2001). Possible medication errors in home healthcare patients. *Journal of the American Geriatrics Society, 49*, 719-724.

Meredith, S., Feldman, P., Frey, D., Giammarco, L., Hall, K., Arnold, K., Brown, N.J., and Ray, W.A. (2002). Improving medication use in home healthcare patients: A randomized controlled trial. *Journal of the American Geriatrics Society, 50*, 1484-1491.

Meredith, S. and Ray, W.A. (1999). Psychotropic drug use in home health care: Problems and directions for research. *Annual Review of Gerontology and Geriatrics, 19,* Chapter 6: (Eds.) Katz, I. & Oslin, D. Springer Publishing Company.

Shaughnessy, P. (2002). Improving patient outcomes of home health care: Findings from two demonstration trials of outcome-based quality improvement. *Journal of the American Geriatrics Society, 50,* 1354-1364.

Title 42–Public Health, Chapter IV, Part 483: Requirements for states and long-term-care facilities. Section 483.25: Quality of care.

Triller, D., Clause, L., Bricelan, L., and Hamilton, R. (2000). Resolution of drug-related problems in home care patients through a pharmacy referral service. *American Journal of Health System Pharmacists, 60(9),* 905-910.

APPENDIX

Home Health Quality Measures

Working with input from measurement experts, the Agency for Healthcare Research and Quality, and a diverse group of home health industry stakeholders, CMS will adopt and publish a set of home health quality measures on every Medicare-certified home health agency in the United States. The 11 quality measures for the Home Health Quality Initiative are a subset of a larger set of OASIS outcome measures that are well known to the home health agencies. They have been extensively tested and studied, and more information on the measures is available at *www.cms.hhs.gov/providers/hha/*. The consumer language below explains the OASIS measures in plain language and will accompany the quality measures found on Home Health Compare at *www.medicare.gov*.

Consumer Language	OASIS Outcome Measure
Patients who get better at getting dressed	Improvement in upper body dressing
Patients who get better at bathing	Improvement in bathing
Patients who stay the same (don't get worse) at bathing	Stabilization in bathing
Patients who get better to and from the toilet	Improvement in toileting
Patients who get better at walking or moving around	Improvement in ambulation/locomotion
Patients who get better at getting in and out of bed	Improvement in transferring
Patients who get better at taking their medications correctly (by mouth)	Improvement in management of oral medications
Patients who are confused less often	Improvement in confusion frequency
Patients who have less pain when moving around	Improvement in pain interfering with activity
Patients who had to be admitted to the hospital	Acute care hospitalization
Patients who need urgent, unplanned medical care	Any emergent care provided

Medication Management Model as Experiential Education Tool for Students of Pharmacy

Darren M. Triller, PharmD

SUMMARY. A visiting nurse association (VNA) and a college of pharmacy sought cost-effective models by which consultant pharmacy services could be offered at a rural branch office to improve medication management for high-risk patients. Through a collaborative relationship with the Albany College of Pharmacy, the Eddy VNA used the structure and support of the Partners in Care Foundation (The Model) Medication Management Model to simultaneously provide patient services and train Doctor of Pharmacy candidates. The Model brings the pharmacist into the homecare team to provide pharmaceutical care and can provide the framework by which pharmacist preceptors and interns can effectively

Darren M. Triller is Assistant Professor, Department of Pharmacy Practice, Albany College of Pharmacy.

Address correspondence to: Darren M. Triller, PharmD, Albany College of Pharmacy, 106 New Scotland Avenue, Albany, NY 12208 (E-mail: trillerd@acp.edu).

The author would like to acknowledge his appreciation for the ongoing support of the staff of the Catskill office of the Eddy VNA, particularly Amber Hurt, RN and Nancy Hadcock, RN.

This project was funded in part by the John A. Hartford Foundation, Inc., New York, New York. The Foundation awarded funding to Partners in Care Foundation to disseminate the Medication Management Model program and to provide technical assistance to leading home health providers across the country, including The Eddy VNA. Project results and toolkit materials can be found at *www.homemeds.org*.

[Haworth co-indexing entry note]: "Medication Management Model as Experiential Education Tool for Students of Pharmacy." Triller, Darren M. Co-published simultaneously in *Home Health Care Services Quarterly* (The Haworth Press, Inc.) Vol. 24, No. 1/2, 2005, pp. 47-59; and: *Improving Medication Management in Home Care: Issues and Solutions* (ed: Dennee Frey) The Haworth Press, Inc., 2005, pp. 47-59. Single or multiple copies of this article are available for a fee from The Haworth Document Delivery Service [1-800-HAWORTH, 9:00 a.m. - 5:00 p.m. (EST). E-mail address: docdelivery@haworthpress.com].

47

provide services to high-risk patients identified through the agency's CQI process. Results from program implementation with 100 Medicaid waiver patients indicate positive staff response and an overall 43% acceptance rate with prescribers and suggest that this is a cost-effective medication management service with implications for adaptation by other HHAs. *[Article copies available for a fee from The Haworth Document Delivery Service: 1-800-HAWORTH. E-mail address: <docdelivery@haworthpress. com> Website: <http://www.HaworthPress.com> © 2005 by The Haworth Press, Inc. All rights reserved.]*

KEYWORDS. Adverse drug event, clerkship, experiential education, home health care, medication management, falls, CQI, pharmacist, consultation

INTRODUCTION

Medical errors have been identified as a national public health problem,[1] and errors relating to the prescription and administration of medications have been identified as a common cause of patient harm in the inpatient and institutional settings.[2] Successful efforts to reduce medication-related errors, drug-related problems (DRPs), and adverse drug events (ADEs) in hospitals have typically involved the active, systematic participation of pharmacists,[3] and higher levels of direct pharmacist involvement in patient care appear to provide greater levels of benefit to patients.[4-6]

While it is possible to facilitate a measure of change in the existing patient care setting, the realities of market forces tend to limit the ability of pharmacists and other care givers to develop and demonstrate the value of novel, non-reimbursed services and programs, especially in settings in which medication management is required yet where traditionally pharmacists are not part of the care team. In contrast, the academic setting is ideal for such activities, as institutions of higher learning are not directly impacted by health care market forces and may also have systems in place to access personnel and fiscal resources necessary for such ventures (e.g., grant funding). In addition, the direct involvement of Doctor of Pharmacy candidates (i.e., pharmacy interns) in such activities makes the involved interns cognizant of the limitations of the existing system, develops problem solving skills, and prepares them for professional practice in the future health care system.

The Medication Management Model[7] is an innovative program that utilizes the active, systematic involvement of pharmacists to reduce adverse drug events and improve patient outcomes in high risk home care recipients. By targeting common and clinically relevant drug-related problems for intervention by pharmacists, the Model has been proven effective in a controlled trial[4] and has been successfully adapted by a variety of home care agencies across the country.[8]

The Catskill office of the Eddy Visiting Nurse Association was a recent recipient of a technical assistance grant to implement the Medication Management Model at the rural agency. In addition to implementing the Model, the agency used the structure and support of the Model, through a collaborative relationship with the Albany College of Pharmacy, to serve as a training tool for pharmacy interns completing clinical rotations in their final year of a Doctor of Pharmacy program. The participation of the college and the students were central to the successful implementation of the Model, and will be important components of the ongoing success of the Model at the agency.

To reduce the adverse impact of DRPS and ADEs in the outpatient setting, changes need to be made in the outpatient medication use system, particularly for high risk home care recipients. Replication of the Medication Management Model, with the active participation of colleges and students of pharmacy, may be an effective means of improving the care provided to home health recipients while simultaneously training the next generation of pharmacists and other health professionals.

PURPOSE

To describe the successful use of the Medication Management Model as a component of an experiential education clerkship at a college of pharmacy and to provide information that may be helpful for successful replication program at other agencies.

SITE DESCRIPTIONS

The Eddy VNA is an affiliate of Northeast Health, a comprehensive, regional network of healthcare and community services. Comprised of The Eddy, Samaritan Hospital and Albany Memorial Hospital, Northeast Health employs more than 4,200 healthcare professionals working at 58 locations throughout the Capital Region. The Eddy VNA, comprised of the predominantly urban Troy office and the rural Catskill office, has been providing care since 1908 and is the largest home health provider in the Capital Region of New York State.

Founded in 1881, Albany College of Pharmacy is the oldest continuously operating pharmacy school in New York State and one of the only private, independent pharmacy schools in the country. The majority of students enrolled in Albany College of Pharmacy pursue a six-year Doctor of Pharmacy degree, with the final year of the program being comprised of five week off-campus clinical clerkship rotations. The present curriculum presently requires students to complete at least one rotation in a community pharmacy, an inpatient facility, and an ambulatory care setting. Students also complete elective rotations in a large variety of other patient care and pharmaceutical industry-related settings.

Institutions within Northeast Health have a longstanding relationship with Albany College of Pharmacy, with Samaritan Hospital and Albany Memorial Hospital participating as practice sites for the institutional pharmacy clerkship program for over 15 years, and NEH's Empire Home Infusion also offers a Home Infusion Pharmacotherapy rotation. In 2000, Albany College of Pharmacy placed the first of five full-time faculty members now practicing within NEH organizations, including the Troy office of the Eddy VNA, Eddy Heritage House Nursing Center, Eddy Cohoes Rehabilitation Center, and two primary care clinics. In addition to course loads and on campus activities, the faculty members act as clinical preceptors at these clinical locations for 12-18 students per year each.

HOME CARE CLINICAL PHARMACY SERVICE

Since the placement of the initial faculty member, the college has assigned students to complete five-week clinical rotations with the faculty at the Troy office of the Eddy VNA HHA. At this Eddy office, the faculty member has developed a referral service[6] by which patients identified by nurses as having difficulty with medication management receive home pharmacist visits. These visits consist of a comprehensive in-home medication assessment which evaluates the drug regimen for all potential drug-related problems and seeks resolution through intervention by the faculty pharmacist and students. This service has demonstrated that DRPs are highly prevalent in the home care population and that pharmacist involvement is an effective means of identifying and resolving such problems. The urban setting and close proximity to the College limits the travel required by faculty and students, and the formal relationship between NEH hospitals and system physician offices facilitates effective communication between the pharmacy personnel and other care providers.

However, the present service,[6] based on the efforts of available faculty and students, provides visits to fewer than 4% of patients at the Troy office of the Eddy VNA, and the service is unable to routinely provide home visits to the patients of the more rural Catskill office, whose patients may be at even greater risk due to geographic isolation and other health care deficiencies in the region. Given these logistical constraints, the VNA and the College sought other models by which a comparable level of pharmacy services could be offered to the patients of the rural Catskill office. Based on previous experiences at the Troy office, it was presumed that the successful model would need to provide valuable clinical services to a significant proportion of patients while simultaneously providing students with a clerkship experience that meets educational outcome objectives and quality requirements of the College.

EDUCATIONAL OUTCOMES

The pharmacy curriculum at the Albany College of Pharmacy is designed to meet specific educational outcome goals, as adopted from the American Association of College of Pharmacy. These *Educational Outcomes*[9] (Table 1) are intended to serve several purposes, the most important of which is to serve as a guide to pharmacy faculty and administrators in assessing and revising their curricula. While each clerkship offering cannot be expected to address every outcome, nonelective clerkships should be effective in addressing some of them, with students demonstrating a level of proficiency in all outcomes prior to graduation.

In considering the activities of the pharmacist involved in the Medication Management Model, it is apparent that several educational objectives would be addressed through active participation of faculty and students in the model. Specifically, the Model intervention brings the pharmacist into the home health care team for the express purpose of providing pharmaceutical care (Outcome I), and provides the framework by which pharmacist and student can effectively provide services. Such structure is essential for the training of students, as it provides detailed guidance to the individual unfamiliar with the practice setting and

TABLE 1. Professional-Based Outcomes[a] (detailed subheadings not included)

I. Provide Pharmaceutical Care
   A. Gather and organize information in order to identify ongoing or potential drug-related problems and the root cause of the problems.
   B. Plan and perform ongoing patient evaluation to identify additional drug-related problems and implement changes in the pharmaceutical care plan.
   C. Interpret and evaluate pharmaceutical data and related information needed to prevent or resolve medication-related problems or to respond to information requests.
   D. Collaborate with physicians, other health care professionals, patients, and/or their caregivers to formulate a pharmaceutical care plan.
   E. Implement the pharmaceutical care plan.
   F. Document pharmaceutical care activity in the patient's medical record to facilitate communication and collaboration among providers.

II. Manage the Practice
   A. Manage Pharmacy Operations
   B. Manage Medication Distribution and Control Systems
   C. Manage Human Resources
   D. Manage Facilities and Equipment
   E. Manage Fiscal Resources
   F. Manage Change in Response to Professional Evolution

III. Manage Medication Use Systems
   A. Participate in the pharmaceutical care system's process for reporting and managing medication errors and adverse drug reactions.
   B. Participate in the pharmaceutical care system's process for conducting drug use evaluations.
   C. Participate in the development, implementation, evaluation, and modification of a formulary system.
   D. Apply principles of outcomes research and quality assessment methods to the evaluation of pharmaceutical care.

IV. Promote Public Health
   A. Provide emergency care on a limited basis.
   B. Promote public awareness of health and disease.

V. Provide Drug Information and Education
   A. Provide pharmaceutical information to health professionals and the general public.
   B. Design, develop, and present educational materials tailored to the needs and educational background of a given audience.

[a]Center for the Advancement of Pharmaceutical Education (CAPE) Advisory Panel on Educational Outcomes. Educational Outcomes. 1998. Accessed at: http://www.aacp.org/site/page.asp?TRACKID= &VID=1&CID=1031&DID=6074 Accessed on: 9/7/2004

assures that a level of homogeneity of experience will be maintained from student to student. The evidence-based Model also provides an excellent example of rational clinical operating procedures that may be helpful in the future development of clinical services in other settings in the graduate's career.

Participation in the Model gives students the opportunity to be involved in control systems (Outcome IIb), and additions to the Model, such as pharmacist/student presentations to patients and staff, can provide opportunities to promote public health and to provide drug information and education (Outcomes IV and V). While such activities are not necessarily part of the formal Model, such interaction between pharmacy and agency personnel may be helpful in fostering professional relationships and increasing the ability of the nursing staff to provide education and medication-related services to their patients. The pharmacy-related activities of the Medication Management Model, therefore, appear to be entirely consistent with the Educational Outcomes of the curriculum of the College, and a useful means of providing clinical student clerkships targeting these outcomes.

CHARACTERISTICS OF A QUALITY CLERKSHIP

In addition to providing activities that are consistent with Educational Outcomes, the College requires that clinical clerkships also meet specific quality characteristics.[10] First, the experience must involve the student in the real-time patient care activities. Hypothetical or virtual patient cases, while not entirely excluded, should not serve as the foundation for the experience. The student activities must contribute to the "real work" of the site, place performance expectations on the student, and provide an experience that is challenging. The highest quality experiences afford the student the opportunity to see their work applied and to observe related patient outcomes. Such activities should be sufficient in quantity to occupy the student's time throughout the assigned rotation period, and students should have constant, although not immediate, access to supervision and have routine scheduled contact with supervisors and clerkship preceptors.

The activities associated with the Medication Management Model meets many of these quality expectations, and site-specific modifications and arrangements can easily be developed to assure that the student receives a quality educational experience. All patient care activities are real, and the contributions of pharmacist and student have direct benefits for the patient and the agency. The student participating in the Model would have the ability to not only identify drug-related problems and to intervene, but to also see the implemented results of their efforts and the impact on the patient. Given a sufficient case load and preceptor and nurse oversight, the Medication Management Model appeared to effectively meet specific Educational Outcomes and provide a high quality educational experience to students of pharmacy.

BENEFITS TO AGENCY

In addition to being a valuable educational tool, the increased presence of pharmacy personnel at the agency has considerable benefits for the patients and staff of the HHA. The clinical benefits to patients have been documented,[4] and the Model clearly enhances quality improvement initiatives relating to medication use. More subtly, the increased availability to nurses of pharmacy information resources increases awareness of medication-related issues, promotes collaborative efforts, and helps foster an environment in which clinical staff is better able to identify and address drug-related problems. Because of its well defined structure and strong supporting evidence, the Model can serve as a bridge that promotes collaboration between clinical and academic institutions, with measurable benefits to be gleaned by both.

IMPLEMENTATION OF MODEL

In the fall of 2002, and with the support of a Technical Assistance Grant from the Partners in Care Foundation, the College and the Catskill office of the Eddy VNA implemented the Medication Management Model as a component of an experiential education offering for students. Students assigned to the Troy office for clerkship were directed to the Catskill office for one full day per week, and the faculty preceptor was scheduled at the Catskill office for the afternoon of the same day. Policies and procedures were developed and the agency staff was oriented to the nature and schedule of the program. In the initial stage the Model was targeted to identify two specific drug-related problems important to the agency's improvement focus and included in the model, duplicative therapies and drugs associated with falls. Other problems identified during case discussions were also acted upon. The program initially targeted patients enrolled in the agency's Long Term Care

(LTC) Program, a 90-patient New York Medicaid carve-out program and any patients for whom an incident report for a fall had been submitted to the administration. The nursing supervisor for the LTC was designated as the liaison between agency and pharmacy, the nursing staff was responsible for obtaining written patient and physician consent for pharmacy services prior to pharmacy accessing private health information.

Students were oriented to the agency during the first week of their assignment, and were charged with initiating patient evaluations during the morning at the office, collecting necessary clinical information from agency records, staff and physician offices as needed (e.g., laboratory results). Upon the weekly arrival of the faculty member, the student, faculty, and nurse supervisor reviewed each case and agreed upon a course of intervention. The student was then responsible for communicating all therapy recommendations to prescribers. If necessary patient-specific details were unavailable, and if the nurse case manager was otherwise engaged, detailed memos were left for the nurse, with the request that the details be provided by the following week. Copies of memos were also directed to the nurse's supervisor to assure a timely response to the request.

Recommendations to prescribers were routinely initiated by telephone contact with the prescriber's office (typically with office nurse), with more detailed recommendations following immediately by fax. It was felt that, due to the often complicated nature of the recommendations, this two-step process was required. A general overview of the issue could easily be provided to a nurse by phone, and the specific written recommendation, including suggestions for changes in orders, could then be faxed to the office for formal presentation to the physician.

In subsequent weeks, students were responsible for follow-up on outstanding recommendations and re-sent to prescribers if necessary. In addition to activities explicit in the Model, students provided a drug-related presentation to the staff each month, and answered drug information questions in person or by phone call to the Troy office throughout the week. The implementation of the Model at the agency in this manner is considered to be both clinically effective for patients and educationally valuable to the students.

RESULTS

Between November 2002 and July 2003 the students provided medication reviews for 100 patients of the agency, with the vast majority

(85) enrolled in the LTC program. The service identified and acted upon 164 drug-related problems with certain patients reporting more than one problem. Forty-five of the generated recommendations were accepted (27%). An additional 26 recommendations were accepted in part (i.e., resulted in some positive action, if not entirely what was recommended), providing an overall response rate of approximately 43%. Although not documented, numerous additional requests for drug information were made of the students, and "curb side" consults were common. Overall, the agency staff was highly receptive to the participation of the pharmacy personnel at the office.

In addition, the Eddy Visiting Nurse Association received a commendation from the Community Health Accreditation Program (CHAP)[a] for medication management, and the faculty pharmacist and clinical staff members were jointly awarded the agency's Very Important Interdepartmental Team Award for 2002 (Troy office) and 2003 (Catskill office). The faculty pharmacist and his research assistant were awarded IPRO's[b] Excellence in Home Health Care Quality Improvement Award in 2003, and the faculty member received the Northeast Health 2003 Golden Torch Award for efforts relating to home care medication management. Such recognition highlights the growing interest in improving medication management of these high risk patients, as well as the high level of acceptance and appreciation of accrediting bodies, peer-review organizations, and health systems for clinical pharmacy services.

Students likewise commented favorably on the experience. All six students completing the rotation in the spring semester of 2003 indicated on exit evaluations that they would recommend the rotation to other students. Reflecting the numerous co-morbidities and complex medication regimens encountered, the opportunity to apply their skills to the evaluation of complicated clinical cases was cited as a strength of the clerkship by four students. Direct exposure to the medication-related problems faced by ambulatory seniors was also cited as a clerkship strength by four students, as traditional retail pharmacy rotations do not necessarily provide this degree of personalized patient perspective. Home visits completed in the Troy office and occasionally in Catskill were also viewed favorably by the students.

DISCUSSION

In addition to being clinically valuable, The Medication Management Model is a highly useful tool for training students of pharmacy.

With only minor alterations and additions to the standard Model, a clinical clerkship rotation may be devised that provides the students with clinical experiences and perspectives not commonly provided in traditional community pharmacy training programs. The successful collaboration between the Eddy and the Albany College of Pharmacy may serve as a model for replication at other home care agencies, especially those near colleges and universities with degree programs in pharmacy. In addition, present trends in the healthcare environment make such collaboration between colleges and agencies more attractive, if not entirely necessary.

A nationwide pharmacist shortage[11] has resulted in a surge in applications to colleges of pharmacy, straining the ability to provide quality clerkship experiences without the identification of new sites or curricular revisions. For example, the enrollment at Albany College of Pharmacy has increased substantially in recent years, with approximately 60 students graduating with the PharmD degrees in 2003 and a projected 150 to 225 in 2006. In addition to the increased numbers of students, the increased focus on pharmaceutical care outcomes in education increases the need for high quality experiences, such as that offered at the Eddy VNA. Therefore, similar agencies located near pharmacy colleges may be well positioned for such collaboration and replication of the Medication Management Model (see Table 2). Agencies interested in such collaboration are encouraged to contact their local college of pharmacy and review materials found on <www.homemeds.org>.

While the present program was successful, it was not without limitations. First, the Model was replicated with the assistance of a pharmacist with previous home care experience. Likewise, the students were not assigned to the single office for the entire clerkship. However, it is the belief of those involved in the present program that the home health rotation Model is well suited for serving as a stand-alone clerkship offering, and the College's Department of Experiential Education is considering means by which this could be accomplished in the immediate future.

For the site to be successful as a stand-alone student site, it is felt that a pharmacist preceptor should be on site at least 8 hours a week (e.g., two half days). The number of patient referrals should be adequate to challenge the students, and strong nurse/staff support in the absence of the pharmacist is necessary. Additional projects, such as educational presentations and joint home visits with nurses, could be added to broaden the student experience and expand the influence of the

TABLE 2. Steps for Agencies Interested in Replicating Model

1. Review Model at web page
2. Identify local colleges of pharmacy
3. Contact dean, college of pharmacy or chair dept pharmacy to discuss
4. Visit college with statistics and info on agency (case load, services, etc.)
5. Discuss curriculum, experiential program and potential needs
6. Discuss potential collaboration based on Med Mgt Model

pharmacy presence at the agency. Likewise, projects and activities at the college (e.g., case presentations, journal club, etc.) may also be employed to enhance the experience for the student.

CONCLUSION

The Medication Management Model is a valuable clinical program that has been shown to improve the care of seniors in a variety of home care settings. By collaborating with a college of pharmacy, home care agencies may find the Medication Management Model to provide a helpful framework for the development of mutually beneficial clinical services and quality improvement activities.

AUTHOR NOTE

Readers are referred to <www.homemeds.org> for additional information about the MMM and to <http://www.aacp.org/site/page.asp?TRACKID=&VID=1&CID=1031&DID=6074> for updated CAPE educational outcomes and of colleges of pharmacy.

NOTES

a. The Community Health Accreditation Program, Inc., 39 Broadway, Suite # 710, New York, NY 10006, (800)656-9656, (212)480-8828, was the first accreditation agency to be recognized (in May 1992) by the Center for Medicare and Medicaid Services (CMS) for Medicare certification of Home Health Care agencies.

b. IPRO, 1979 Marcus Avenue, Lake Success, NY 11042-1002, is one of the nation's largest and most experienced health care evaluation and quality improvement organizations. An independent, not-for-profit New York corporation, IPRO's clients include federal and state agencies, providers, managed care organizations, commercial insurers, Fortune 500 companies, business coalitions and unions across the country.

REFERENCES

1. Kohn, L.T., Corrigan, J.M., & Donaldson, M.D. (Eds.) (1999). *To err is human: Building a safer health system.* Washington, DC: National Academy Press.

2. Institute of Medicine (U.S.) (2003). Committee on Quality of Health Care in America. Priority Areas for National Action: Transforming Health Care Quality. The National Academy Press.

3. Leape, L.L., Cullen, D.J., Clapp, M.D. et al. (1999). Pharmacist participation on physician rounds and adverse drug events in the intensive care unit. *JAMA, 282,* 267-270.

4. Meredith, S., Feldman, P., Frey, D. et al. (2002). Improving medication use in newly admitted home healthcare patients: A randomized controlled trial. *Journal of the American Geriatric Society, 50,* 1484-1491.

5. Stewart, S., Vandenbroek, A.J., Pearson, S., & Horowitz, J.D. (1999). Prolonged beneficial effects of a home-based intervention on unplanned readmissions and mortality among patients with congestive heart failure. *Archives of Internal Medicine, 159,* 257-261.

6. Triller, D.M., Clause, S.L., Briceland, L.L., & Hamilton, R.A. (2003). Resolution of drug-related problems in home care patients. *American Journal of Health System Pharmacy, 60,* 905-910.

7. Brown, N.J., Griffin, M.R., Ray, W.A. et al. (1998). A model for improving medication use in home health care patients. *Journal of the American Pharmacy Association, 38*(6), 696-702.

8. Frey, D., & Rahman, A. (2003). Medication management: An evidence-based model that decreases adverse events. *Home Healthcare Nurse, 21*(6), 404-412.

9. Center for the Advancement of Pharmaceutical Education (CAPE) Advisory Panel on Educational Outcomes. Educational Outcomes. 1998. Accessed at: http://www.aacp.org/Docs/MainNavigation/Resources/3933_ edoutcom.doc?DocTypeID=4&TrackID=&VID=1&CID=410&DID=366. Accessed on: November 24, 2003.

10. Carter, J.T., Draugalis, J.R., & Slack, M.K. (1996). Impact of clerkship students on pharmacy-site output. *American Journal of Health System Pharmacy, 53,* 1694-1700.

11. Knapp, K.K., & Livesey, J.C. (2002). The Aggregate Demand Index: Measuring the balance between pharmacist supply and demand, 1999-2001. *Journal of the American Pharmacy Association, 42,* 391-398.

Reaching the Homebound Elderly:
The Prescription Intervention
and Lifelong Learning (PILL) Program

Bradley R. Williams, PharmD, FASCP, CGP
Suzanna Lopez, PharmD, CGP

SUMMARY. This article describes the Prescription Intervention and Lifelong Learning (PILL) program, a three-year pilot project to develop in-home pharmacy care services to clients of a community-based social service agency. Clients who were homebound, at least 62 years of age, and taking at least five medications were eligible for inclusion. Potential participants were referred by care managers to the pharmacist, who conducted an in-home evaluation of the medication regimen and assessed the risk for medication-related problems. The pharmacist provided instruction for hypertension and diabetes mellitus self-monitoring, extensive medication counseling for clients with complex medications regimens, and conducted other activities to promote positive medica-

Bradley R. Williams is Professor, Clinical Pharmacy and Clinical Gerontology at University of Southern California, School of Pharmacy, 1985 Zonal Avenue, PSC 110, Andrus Gerontology Center, Los Angeles, CA 90089-9121 (E-mail: bradwill@usc.edu). Suzanna Lopez is Clinical Pharmacist with Comprehensive Pharmacy Services, Los Angeles, CA (E-mail: pillpharm@hotmail.com).

This project was supported, in part, by a grant from the Archstone Foundation. The authors gratefully acknowledge the efforts of the staff of the Southeast Area Social Services Funding Authority (SASSFA), who were an integral part of the program. Nancy Vong assisted with the data management for the project.

[Haworth co-indexing entry note]: "Reaching the Homebound Elderly: The Prescription Intervention and Lifelong Learning (PILL) Program." Williams, Bradley R., and Suzanna Lopez. Co-published simultaneously in *Home Health Care Services Quarterly* (The Haworth Press, Inc.) Vol. 24, No. 1/2, 2005, pp. 61-72; and: *Improving Medication Management in Home Care: Issues and Solutions* (ed: Dennee Frey) The Haworth Press, Inc., 2005, pp. 61-72. Single or multiple copies of this article are available for a fee from The Haworth Document Delivery Service [1-800-HAWORTH, 9:00 a.m. - 5:00 p.m. (EST). E-mail address: docdelivery@haworthpress.com].

tion-related outcomes. The clients served were primarily female, between 70 and 90 years of age, and almost one-half lived alone. They were taking an average of more than nine medications daily, and had at least one chronic disease. The clients of the social service agency were highly vulnerable to medication-related problems and were in need of in-home pharmacy care services. *[Article copies available for a fee from The Haworth Document Delivery Service: 1-800-HAWORTH. E-mail address: <docdelivery@haworthpress.com> Website: <http://www.HaworthPress.com>* © 2005 by The Haworth Press, Inc. All rights reserved.]

KEYWORDS. Home health care, medication-related problems, elderly, pharmacist interventions, geriatric drug use

The geriatric population constitutes the fastest rising segment of the U.S. population (Day, 1996) and is a major consumer of health care services, including medications. While the effects of the proposed Medicare prescription drug benefit are not yet known, it is likely that it will significantly increase government expenditures for medications (Heffler et al., 2004). Currently, people age 65 years and older comprise 12.4% of the total U.S. population; this percentage is expected to increase to nearly 20% by 2030 (Day JC, 1996). This represents a growth rate of 58% over 30 years and reflects both the aging of the baby boom generation and an increase in overall life expectancy.

Increased longevity, however, is not necessarily accompanied by good health. Nearly 30% of older adults consider their health status to be fair or poor. Some disability is present in over 30% of people age 65-74, and in almost 45% of people aged 75 and above (Blackwell et al., 2003). Arthritis, hypertension, respiratory illnesses, heart disease, diabetes, stroke, and cancer are the most common chronic conditions encountered among the elderly (Adams et al., 1999). Perceived poor health status, disability, and multiple disease states lead to higher health care costs and use of a greater number of medications (Moxey, 2003).

The expanding geriatric population has created a need for effective methods to manage the health care of frail elderly in a non-institutional setting. Elderly people, the majority of whom live at home, take a wide range of medications to manage their chronic diseases. More than 58% take cardiovascular system drugs and over 28% take analgesics. Antidepressants, tranquilizers, and similar medications are taken by 18% of the nation's elderly. Anti-seizure and muscle relaxing agents are taken by 13% of older adults (Moxey, 2003).

This widespread medication use by older adults increases the likelihood for medication-related problems (MRP). Compounding the risk for MRP are physiological changes that affect drug behavior in the body, multiple medical conditions, social isolation, and fragmented health care. Despite the knowledge that medications can cause significant problems for the elderly, more than one in five of community-dwelling older adults receive medications that are considered potentially inappropriate (Beers, 1997; Curtis, 2004). It has been estimated that 25% of hospital admissions for people age 65 and older are related to medications, with polypharmacy, adverse drug reactions and noncompliance being the primary causes (Col et al.,1990; Flaherty et al., 2000).

Home care has enabled many older adults to remain at home while recovering from serious illness or to receive skilled nursing and rehabilitation services over extended periods of time without having to reside in a hospital or nursing facility. However, home care often is time limited, and may not serve the needs of permanently frail or disabled older adults.

Many frail elders who live at home receive care management from senior centers or other agencies. Services provided typically include social services, home-delivered meals, and coordination of medical appointments. Many clients of care management organizations may be medically frail and take several medications; up to one-third of home healthcare clients may be taking medications that are inappropriate for their age or condition (Meredith et al., 2001). There is no widely available system for managing pharmacotherapy and typically no available expertise regarding the appropriate use of medications in this population; nor is there any mechanism for routine reimbursement for provision of such services.

Pharmacists have provided consultative services to home health agencies for more than twenty years. Coleman et al. (1982) reviewed the medication use patterns among 95 clients of a visiting nurse association (VNA). Clients were taking an average of 8.4 medications. Nonadherence (62%), improper medication storage (35%), duplicate medications (8%) and inappropriate doses (8%) were the most common problems noted during home visits. Following the completion of the study, the VNA incorporated a pharmacist into its organization and sustained the service for well over a decade. The pharmacist continued to review medications and intervene with health care providers, clients, and families (Frey, 1986; Frey, 1987).

A randomized, controlled study of a pharmacist's intervention for one year in a home health agency was conducted by Williams et al.

(1987). Among those receiving the pharmacist intervention, duplicate medications and the prescribing of medications without a diagnosis decreased; the average number of medications per patient increased.

Zuckerman et al. (1986) offered drug information services, home visits, educational programs, and participated in hospice and patient care conferences at a home health agency in Baltimore. A pharmacist intervention was required for 38/288 (19%) of patients newly admitted to the service. The pharmacist made eight home visits and responded to an additional 60 requests for drug information. As a result of the pilot project, a pharmacist was added to the agency's board of directors and a long-term service contract was implemented.

Economic factors associated with pharmacist services were investigated during a 12-month study conducted in a home health agency (Ryan et al., 1988). Working in collaboration with a physician and home health nurse, the pharmacist reduced drug utilization by 27% among 840 homebound patients. The pharmacists' recommendations to prescribers were implemented in 72% of the instances. A drug cost savings of over $183,000, or approximately $218/patient in 1988 dollars, was realized.

A hospital-based in-home medication evaluation by a pharmacist was conducted at a Veterans' Administration hospital. Initial home visits to 20 elderly patients noted potentially unnecessary medication in the home (70%), drugs taken incorrectly (60%) or not taken at all (55%), expired medications (35%) and other medication-related problems. Pharmacist interventions led to significant ($p < 0.05$) reductions in medication discrepancies, the presence of unnecessary drugs, and expired medications (Hsia-Der et al., 1997).

The largest investigation of pharmacist services to a home health agency was conducted in two large, urban agencies (Meredith et al., 2002). The two-year, parallel-group, randomized controlled trial focused on four problem areas, unnecessary therapeutic duplication, cardiovascular medications, potentially inappropriate use of psychotropic medications, and the use of non-steroidal anti-inflammatory drugs (NSAID) in patients with a high risk for peptic ulcer complications. The pharmacist served as a consultant to the home health agency nurses. The use of unnecessary medications was significantly reduced ($p = 0.003$) and cardiovascular medication use was improved ($p = 0.017$).

Ongoing monitoring of drug therapy, however, typically stops when the client is discharged from the home health service. Consequently, frail elders living at home generally do not receive long-term monitoring of their frequently complex medication regimens.

The Prescription Intervention and Lifelong Learning (PILL) program was developed as a project to demonstrate the potential value of consultant pharmacist services to homebound elderly clients who received care management services from a community social services agency. PILL was a three-year, community health promotion project designed to assist local communities in obtaining integrative pharmaceutical care services and medication education directed toward homebound elderly. The primary goal was to assist older adults to live as independently as possible and to avoid unnecessary hospitalization or institutionalization. This report describes the PILL program and provides an overview of the population served.

METHODS

PILL was a comprehensive medication management pilot program designed to assist homebound senior citizens and their caregivers. A pharmacist trained in geriatric pharmacotherapy was employed to conduct medication evaluations in the client's home. The program was approved by the investigational review board (IRB) at Los Angeles County/USC Medical Center (LAC+USCMC). Informed consent was obtained from potential subjects prior to their inclusion in the program.

Eligibility to receive PILL services was determined by the following criteria:

- Client of the Southeast Area Social Services Funding Authority (SASSFA) in southeast Los Angeles County
- Homebound as determined by SASSFA eligibility criteria
- At least 60 years of age
- Taking 5 or more prescription and/or non-prescription medications

Program flow for clients receiving SASSFA services is shown in Figure 1. Following an initial referral to an intake worker, a potential client was evaluated by a care manager for eligibility to receive home care services. Those meeting the eligibility criteria for the PILL program were referred to the pharmacist; those requiring nutrition services were referred to a dietitian. A home visit was made to eligible clients by a SASSFA care manager for a home care needs assessment. After informed consent was obtained for participation in the program, the pharmacist visited the client for an in-home evaluation. (SASSFA clients provided written informed consent to receive general program services.

FIGURE 1. PILL Program Flow

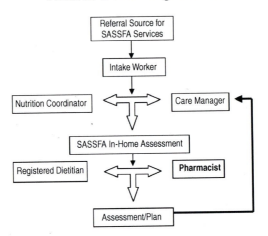

A separate verbal consent was obtained from clients for inclusion in the PILL program. Clients who refused to participate in the study portion continued to receive services, but their information was not included in the study database.)

During the home visit, the pharmacist recorded all medication information (drug name, strength, directions for use, storage method, dose count). The pharmacist also assessed the client's understanding of each medication and its indication, ability to read the prescription label and functional ability, e.g., opening the container and whether the client required assistance with medications. Demographic information, medical information (diseases, health care providers, etc.) and daily function assessment were obtained from SASSFA records maintained for participation in other care management programs (e.g., in-home assistance, home delivered meals).

The pharmacist's assessment included collection of both medication history and use patterns. Following the pharmacist's assessment, an individualized care plan was designed. The care plan was dependent on the medical condition, social need, medication-related problems, goals of therapy, patient cooperation, pharmacist intervention, follow-up and monitoring. The pharmacist assisted a large number of clients with medication management, i.e., organization, compliance issues, drug identification, etc. Similarly, the pharmacist provided medication regimen review, extensive counseling, improving basic knowledge of diseases and medications, and monitoring. Disease management training (e.g., self-monitoring blood sugar and blood pressure) was provided to the patient and caregivers. Additional services included, but were not limited to, referral to other services, communication with primary health care providers and insurance carriers.

RESULTS

Over 150 clients were eligible for inclusion in the program. The pharmacist visited and followed a total of 71 clients. Clients were seen based on the severity of potential medication-related problems; not all eligible clients were seen, due to limited resources. The demographic characteristics of the eligible PILL population are shown in Table 1.

Clients typically reported suffering from multiple chronic medical conditions. Every client was treated for at least one chronic disorder. The 10 most commonly encountered diseases or conditions are listed in Table 2.

The average number of medications taken daily for all clients at entry into the program was 9.62 (range 5-31). The total included both prescription and non-prescription drugs. Many of the medications were considered to be potentially harmful to older adults, as determined by the criteria for potentially inappropriate medications developed by Beers et al. (1997). Table 3 includes the potentially inappropriate medications most commonly prescribed for clients upon entry into the PILL program.

The pharmacist conducted 132 home visits among 71 clients who were seen. The most common interventions made by the pharmacist were monitoring of blood pressure and/or blood glucose, patient counseling regarding appropriate medication use, contacting the physician and/or dispensing pharmacist about a potential medication-related problem, and referring a client to an integrated care management program. Other services included recommending medication-related laboratory tests, disposing of expired prescription medications, helping clients obtain financial assistance for medications (e.g., drug manufacturer-sponsored assistance programs), and referring clients to nutrition or home-delivered meals programs.

Outcomes data are being analyzed and will be reported in a future article.

TABLE 1. Demographics of PILL Population (N = 150)

Characteristic	%
Age (Mean = 78.5 years Range = 63-99 years)	
60-69	6.6
70-79	43.3
80-89	35.3
90-99	14.7
Female Gender	71
Ethnicity	
White-Non-Hispanic	60.3
African-American	0.6
American Indian/Native Alaskan	1.2
Hispanic	37.3
Asian/Pacific Islander	0.6
Living Alone	41.3
Adult Protective Services (APS) Cases	22.4

TABLE 2. Most Common Chronic Conditions Among the PILL Clients (N = 150)

Condition	Number Reporting
Hypertension	65
Diabetes mellitus	45
Osteoarthritis	34
Congestive heart failure	20
Urinary incontinence	19
Hypothyroidism	18
Angina	18
Hypercholesterolemia	17
Constipation	17
Depression	16

DISCUSSION

The clients enrolled in the PILL program were frail individuals who are aging in place. The average age of clients was 78.5 years of age and

TABLE 3. Potentially Inappropriate Medications Prescribed to PILL Clients (N = 150)

Potentially Inappropriate Medication	Number Receiving
Digoxin (> 0.25 mg/day)	23
Sedating antihistamines	13
Long-acting benzodiazepine	12
Tricyclic antidepressants	12
Propoxyphene	9
Anticholinergic medications	8
Propranolol	6
Muscle relaxants	4

the majority suffered from chronic diseases that in general reflect the patterns of disease among the elderly U.S. population (Adams et al., 1999). Most were female, 40% lived alone, and 22% were adult protective service clients. Thus, the elders served constituted a vulnerable population at risk for negative health outcomes.

Medication use was high among the sample. An average of 9.6 medications is well above the norm for community-dwelling elderly (Moxey, 2003), and many were taking in excess of 20 medications daily. Attempting to manage multiple medications predisposes the older adult to adverse drug reactions, drug interactions, and non-adherence. All of those factors increase the risk for drug-induced hospitalizations (Col et al., 1990; Flaherty et al., 2000).

Instruction for home monitoring of blood pressure or blood glucose was the most frequent activity performed by the pharmacist. This reflects both the prevalence of hypertension and diabetes mellitus among PILL clients and the lack of education that they receive from their health care providers. Self-monitoring not only provides a record that can be evaluated by the physician, it also helps to remind the patient of the importance of therapy and to immediately observe how well the disease is controlled.

Providing medication education and counseling was the second most frequent service provided by the pharmacist. In-home education serves as a necessary supplement to information that may be provided by a prescriber or dispensing pharmacist. A patient who visits multiple physicians or who purchases medications at multiple pharmacies may never see a clinician who can see and review all medications and other remedies taken by that patient. Consequently, potential drug-drug, -disease, -food, or -laboratory interactions may never be appropriately evaluated. The in-home visit also ensures that the pharmacist can observe the patient's living environment and medication storage practices, and can spend the necessary time to provide complete and appropriate guidance for medication use.

Older adults who are not educated about their medications or are confused may not be comfortable approaching a health care professional with questions. Many older adults may be reluctant to ask questions because they do not want to challenge the authority of the prescribing physician. The pharmacist was able to identify potential problems of which the client was unaware and to serve as the patient advocate to the prescriber or dispensing pharmacist. In addition, when necessary medication was not taken because the patient could not afford it, the pharmacist was able to assist the client in obtaining the medication through an assistance program.

The use of potentially inappropriate medications was common among the client sample, which is consistent with results from other investigators (Coleman et al., 1982; Golden et al., 1999; Meredith et al., 2001). The most commonly encountered inappropriate medication was digoxin in a dose above 0.25 mg daily. Most of the other agents encountered present a high risk for sedation, dizziness, or falls. Many, including the sedating antihistamines, tricyclic antidepressants, anticholinergic agents, and muscle relaxants, predispose older adults to dry mouth, constipation, urine retention, and blurred vision; at higher doses they can cause confusion and delirium. All increase the risk for significant adverse effects; safer, and possibly more effective alternatives exist (Beers, 1997). Whether the frequency of their use in this group of people is the result of inattention or inexperience on the part of prescribing and dispensing health professionals, of medication formulary restrictions, or some other factor, is yet to be determined. The continuing persistence of this among all elderly populations, however, is of great concern (Curtis et al., 2004).

Providing all of the PILL program services required about 70% full-time effort on the part of the pharmacist (SL). The salary and fringe benefits were paid for from a grant received by the Southeast Area Social Services Funding Authority (SASSFA). Agency overhead was not sufficient to continue the program beyond the length of the pilot project. Because SASSFA serves a low- to lower-middle income clientele and services are not covered by Medicare, Medicaid, or private insurance, potential clients were unable to afford the service, despite the potential benefits. Of note is that during the project two large managed care organizations (MCO) became aware that some of their elderly enrollees were receiving PILL services. Representatives from each MCO conducted a site visit and inquired about having other enrollees participate in the program. When discussions turned to payment by the MCO for the services provided by the program, the organizations declined to participate.

It is clear that there is a population of frail, homebound elderly who can benefit from in-home pharmacist services. Evaluation of medication appropriateness, assistance with therapy self-monitoring, patient education, and intervention on behalf of the patient with health professionals are activities that appropriately-trained pharmacists are well qualified to provide. Two factors that must be addressed in order for this to become a common practice are demonstration of positive therapeutic and economic outcomes, and a mechanism for reimbursement for services.

REFERENCES

Adams, P.F., Hendershot, G.E., & Marano, M.A. (1999). Current estimates from the National Health Interview Survey. 1996. National Center for Health Statistics. *Vital Health Statistics, 10*(200).

Beers, M.H. (1997). Explicit criteria for determining potentially inappropriate medication use by the elderly. *Archvies Internal Medicine, 157*(14),1531-1536.

Blackwell, D.L., & Tonthat, L. (2003). Summary health statistics for the U. S. population: National Health Interview Survey, 1999. National Center for Health Statistics. *Vital Health Stat., 10*(211).

Col, N., Fanale, J.E., & Kronholm, P. (1990). The role of medication noncompliance and adverse drug reactions in hospitalization of the elderly. *Archives Internal Medicine, 150*(4), 841-845.

Coleman, L., Williams, B., & Roth, S. (1982). Description of drug utilization patterns in a home health care setting. *Calif Pharmacist, 30*(4), 26-30.

Curtis, L.H., Østbye, T., Sendersky, V. et al. (2004). Inappropriate prescribing for elderly Americans in a large outpatient population. *Arch Intern Med, 164*(15),1621-1625.

Day, J.C. (1996). Population projections of the United States by age, race, sex and Hispanic origin: 1995 to 2050. U.S. Bureau of the Census, *Current Population Reports*, P25-1130, U.S. Government Printing Office, Washington, DC.

Flaherty, J.H., Perry, H.M., & Lynchard, G.S. et al. (2000). Polypharmacy and hospitalization among older home care patients. *Journal of Gerontology: Med Sci, 55A*(10), M554-M559.

Frey, D. (1986). Pharmacology Assistance Program. Presented at the National Association for Home Care Annual Meeting September. 9-13, 1986.

Frey, D. (1987). Pharmacology Assistance Program–Cost Effectiveness and Evaluation (Abstract) Presented at the National Association for Home Care Annual Meeting, October 10-14, 1987.

Golden, A.G., Preston, R.A., & Barnett, S.D. et al. (1999). Inappropriate medication prescribing in homebound elderly. *Journal of American Geriatric Society, 47*(8), 948-953.

Heffler, S., Smith, S., & Keehan, S. et al. (2004). Health spending projections through 2013. *Health Affairs*, Web Exclusive <http://content.healthaffairs.org/cgi/content/abstract/hlthaff.w4.79>.

Hsia-Der, E., Rubenstein, L.Z., & Choy, G.S. (1997). The benefits of in-home pharmacy evaluation for older persons. *Journal of American Geriatric Society, 45*(2), 211-214.

Meredith, S., Feldman, P.H., Frey, D. et al. (2001). Possible medication errors in home healthcare patients. *J Am Geriatr Soc, 49*(6), 719-724.

Meredith, S., Feldman, P., & Frey, D. et al. (2002). Improving medication use in newly admitted home healthcare patients: A randomized controlled trial. *Journal American Geriatric Society, 50*(9), 1484-1491.

Moxey, E.D., O'Connor, J.P., & Novielli, K.D. et al. (2003). Prescription drug use in the elderly: A descriptive analysis. *Health Care Financing Review, 24*(2), 127-141.

Ryan, P.B., Rush, D.R., Dodd, K.F. et al. (1988). Cost-effective drug regimen review program for home health care patients. *Home Health Service Quarterly, 9*(4), 5-18.

Williams, R.G., McCoy, R., & Frederick, K.R. (1987). Impact of pharmacy consultant services to a homebound population. *Consulting Pharmacology, 2*(6), 479-482.

Zuckerman, I.H., Feinberg, M., Kerr, R.A. et al. (1986). Consultant pharmacy services to a home health care agency. *Consulting Pharmacology, 1*(2), 123-128.

Comment
on Medication Management Models and Other Pharmacist Interventions: Implications for Policy and Practice

Kathleen A. Cameron, RPh, MPH

SUMMARY. Implementation of the Medicare Modernization Act (MMA) of 2003 poses challenges for policy makers and administrators, not the least of which is a provision that high-risk or "targeted" beneficiaries receive Medication Therapy Management (MTM) Services. To ensure that Congressional intent is carried out when Medicare Part D goes into effect in January 2006, the Centers for Medicare & Medicaid Services (CMS) is responsible for issuing regulations to operationalize MTM Services. This article comments on the policy and practice implications of providing such services, including recommendations of the American Society of Consultant Pharmacists (ASCP) and presents findings from the Medication Management Model and other community-based pharmacist-centered interventions as examples of solutions to improve medication

Kathleen A. Cameron is Executive Director for America's Senior Care Pharmacists (ASCP), Research & Education Foundation, Alexandria, Virginia.

Address correspondence to: Kathleen A. Cameron, RPh, MPH, Executive Director, America's Senior Care Pharmacists (ASCP), Research and Education Foundation, 1321 Duke Street, Alexandria, VA 22314 (E-mail: <kcameron@ascp.com> or <www.ascpfoundation. org>).

[Haworth co-indexing entry note]: "Comment on Medication Management Models and Other Pharmacist Interventions: Implications for Policy and Practice." Cameron, Kathleen A. Co-published simultaneously in *Home Health Care Services Quarterly* (The Haworth Press, Inc.) Vol. 24, No. 1/2, 2005, pp. 73-85; and: *Improving Medication Management in Home Care: Issues and Solutions* (ed: Dennee Frey) The Haworth Press, Inc., 2005, pp. 73-85. Single or multiple copies of this article are available for a fee from The Haworth Document Delivery Service [1-800-HAWORTH, 9:00 a.m. - 5:00 p.m. (EST). E-mail address: docdelivery@haworthpress.com].

management and prevent medication-related problems in Medicare beneficiaries. *[Article copies available for a fee from The Haworth Document Delivery Service: 1-800-HAWORTH. E-mail address: <docdelivery@haworthpress.com> Website: <http://www.HaworthPress.com> © 2005 by The Haworth Press, Inc. All rights reserved.]*

KEYWORDS. Medication Therapy Management, Medicare Modernization Act, pharmacist services, home health

Implementation of the Medicare Modernization Act (MMA) of 2003 poses many challenges for policy makers and administrators, not the least of which is a provision that high-risk or "targeted" beneficiaries receive Medication Therapy Management (MTM) Services (Figure 1). To ensure that Congressional intent is carried out when Medicare Part D goes into effect in January 2006, the Centers for Medicare & Medicaid Services (CMS) is responsible for issuing regulations to operationalize MTM Services. Since the MMA legislation was passed, the American Society of Consultant Pharmacists (ASCP) addressed many of these regulatory issues in Issue Briefs, which can be accessed through ASCP's *Medicare Pharmacy Benefit Briefing Room* at <www.ascp.com/Medicare Rx/>. Much of this commentary is based on these Issue Briefs.

Currently several key policy-related questions must be answered prior to the implementation of MTM Services:

- How are the targeted beneficiaries defined?
- Who may authorize the provision of MTM Services to the targeted beneficiaries?
- What is the definition of MTM services?
- Who may provide these MTM Services?
- How will CMS ensure that MTM Services are delivered to the Medicare beneficiaries who need them?

Pharmacist interventions, such as the Home Health Medication Management Model developed by the Partners in Care Foundation, serve as relevant and useful models from which to answer these key policy and regulatory questions. The Medication Management Model consisted of advice from a consultant pharmacist to the attending nurse based on guidelines developed for this intervention. The clinical trial of this model demonstrated that medication errors can be avoided and pre-

FIGURE 1. Medication Therapy Management Services

(c) COST AND UTILIZATION MANAGEMENT; QUALITY ASSURANCE; MEDICATION THERAPY MANAGEMENT PROGRAM–

(1) IN GENERAL–The PDP sponsor shall have in place, directly or through appropriate arrangements, with respect to covered part D drugs, the following:

(A) A cost-effective drug utilization management program, including incentives to reduce costs when medically appropriate, such as through the use of multiple source drugs (as defined in section 41927(k)(7)(A)(i)).

(B) Quality assurance measures and systems to reduce medication errors and adverse drug interactions and improve medication use.

(C) A medication therapy management program described in paragraph (2).

(D) A program to control fraud, abuse, and waste.

Nothing in this section shall be construed as impairing a PDP sponsor from utilizing cost management tools (including differential payments) under all methods of operation.

(2) MEDICATION THERAPY MANAGEMENT PROGRAM–

(A) DESCRIPTION–

(i) IN GENERAL–A medication therapy management program described in this paragraph is a program of drug therapy management that may be furnished by a pharmacist and that is designed to assure, with respect to targeted beneficiaries described in clause (ii), that covered part D drugs under the prescription drug plan are appropriately used to optimize therapeutic outcomes through improved medication use, and to reduce the risk of adverse events, including adverse drug interactions. Such a program may distinguish between services in ambulatory and institutional settings.

(ii) TARGETED BENEFICIARIES DESCRIBED–Targeted beneficiaries described in this clause are part D eligible individuals who–

(I) have multiple chronic diseases (such as diabetes, asthma, hypertension, hyperlipidemia, and congestive heart failure);

(II) are taking multiple covered part D drugs; and

(III) are identified as likely to incur annual costs for covered part D drugs that exceed a level specified by the Secretary.

(B) ELEMENTS–Such program may include elements that promote–

(i) enhanced enrollee understanding to promote the appropriate use of medications by enrollees and to reduce the risk of potential adverse events associated with medications, through beneficiary education, counseling, and other appropriate means;

(ii) increased enrollee adherence with prescription medication regimens through medication refill reminders, special packaging, and other compliance programs and other appropriate means; and

(iii) detection of adverse drug events and patterns of overuse and underuse of prescription drugs.

(C) DEVELOPMENT OF PROGRAM IN COOPERATION WITH LICENSED PHARMACISTS–Such program shall be developed in cooperation with licensed and practicing pharmacists and physicians.

FIGURE 1 (continued)

(D) COORDINATION WITH CARE MANAGEMENT PLANS–The Secretary shall establish guidelines for the coordination of any medication therapy management program under this paragraph with respect to a targeted beneficiary with any care management plan established with respect to such beneficiary under a chronic care improvement program under section 1807.

(E) CONSIDERATIONS IN PHARMACY FEES–The PDP sponsor of a prescription drug plan shall take into account, in establishing fees for pharmacists and others providing services under such plan, the resources used, and time required to, implement the medication therapy management program under this paragraph. Each such sponsor shall disclose to the Secretary upon request the amount of any such management or dispensing fees. The provisions of section 1927(b)(3)(D) apply to information disclosed under this subparagraph.

scribing practices can be improved in this vulnerable population: Medication use improved in 50% of intervention patients, compared to 38% of controls (p = .05) (Meredith et al., 2002). There was no evidence of adverse intervention effects, e.g., new medication problems, more agency nurse visits, or increased duration of home health care.

The Medication Management Model was replicated in four sites in three states–New York, California, and West Virginia–that encompass rural, urban, and suburban settings. The home health agencies, which include both for-profit and not-for-profit entities, have adapted the Medication Management Model using innovative approaches that are specific to their agencies and the needs of their clientele.

The model now is being tested in California's Multi-Purpose Senior Services Program (MSSP), a Medicaid home and community-based waiver program serving frail low income seniors, as a grantee of the Administration on Aging (AoA) Evidence-based Prevention programs. AoA, part of the U.S. Department of Health and Human Services (HHS), in 2003 awarded grants totaling over $2 million as part of a public/private partnership to increase access for older people to programs that have proven to be effective in reducing the risk of disease, injury, and disability. The partnership involves a variety of federal agencies and private foundations that are coordinating their efforts to help implement evidence-based prevention programs through aging services providers at the community level. Medication management is one of the key focus areas of this important initiative.

Another example of an effective pharmacist intervention program is Senior PHARM*Assist* located in Durham County, North Carolina which since 1994 has assisted senior adults, 65 years and older, to obtain medicines they need and avoid ones they don't. The goal is to help seniors with limited incomes remain as healthy and independent as possible, thus remaining out of institutions and in their own homes. Medication reviews are provided for each participant. Every six months, each participant meets with a program pharmacist for one-on-one counseling to talk about correct and safe medication use and other preventive health practices. The pharmacist encourages adherence to prescribed medication schedules and instructions and reviews current medications to identify potential problems. Each senior receives a medication record listing all of his/her medications and is encouraged to maintain the record and share it with other health care providers.

Senior PHARM*Assist* is recognized across the state and nation as a model for pharmaceutical care for older adults. After participating in the program for one year, nearly one-third fewer participants used emergency rooms and stayed overnight in hospitals (Upchurch et al., 2001). This innovative program demonstrates that helping seniors learn about community resources and obtain necessary medicines, while avoiding unnecessary ones, is improving lives.

These projects, as well as the many community-based pharmacist run medication management programs around the country, must be examined by CMS as MTM services are defined, developed and implemented. (Note: For additional information about model programs, the reader is referred to ASCP's monthly journal, *The Consultant Pharmacist* which has featured several of these pharmacist programs since 1999).

DEFINITION OF TARGETED BENEFICIARIES

The Medicare Modernization Act defines targeted beneficiaries as Part D eligible individuals who:

- have multiple chronic diseases, such as diabetes, asthma, hypertension, hyperlipidemia, and congestive heart failure;
- are taking multiple covered Medicare Part D drugs; and
- are identified as likely to incur annual costs for covered Part D drugs that exceed a level specified by the Secretary of Health and Human Services.

Medicare beneficiaries with multiple chronic conditions are especially likely to be clients of home health agencies; Medicaid home and community-based waiver programs, such as PACE (Program of All-inclusive Care for the Elderly), MSSP and Adult day service centers; and assisted living residents.

CMS will "set the bar" with regard to how many Medicare beneficiaries qualify to receive these services. Should the bar be set high or low? The ASCP Research and Education Foundation's Fleetwood Project considered this question when the "Fleetwood Model" was developed in 1997. Although applied only in nursing facilities currently, the Fleetwood Model consists of a prospective and retrospective pharmacist intervention for residents at highest risk for medication-related problems, direct communication with prescribers, and assessment by the pharmacist.

The first step in developing the Fleetwood Model was the identification of factors that place frail, elderly nursing facility residents at highest risk for medication-related problems (see Table 1).

Several assumptions led to the development of this high risk factor algorithm. Not all patients experience preventable medication-related problems that result in costly negative outcomes. In addition, it is not feasible or reasonable to provide pharmaceutical care to all patients receiving medications, nor are payers likely to pay for this level of pharmacist services for everyone. Focusing on patients at highest risk for medication-related problems that result in the most costly negative outcomes allows pharmacists and other health care professionals to more efficiently and economically focus their attention on those seniors with the greatest need and who may realize the greatest benefit.

Another critical factor to be considered when "setting the bar" is that the supply of pharmacists and other health professionals with expertise in geriatric drug therapy is limited. For example, only about 1,000 pharmacists have qualified to be credentialed as Certified Geriatric Pharmacists by the Commission for Certification in Geriatric Pharmacy.

AUTHORIZING MTM SERVICES

Once the criteria for MTM Services are defined, who authorizes the provision of MTM Services to the targeted beneficiaries? Since the Prescription Drug Plans (PDPs) are required in the legislation to provide medication therapy management services as well as disease management and quality assurance services, they are obviously able to autho-

TABLE 1. Risk Factors for Medication-Related Problems Among Elderly Nursing Facility Residents

Specific Medication
Digoxin
Warfarin
Lithium
Theophylline
Chlorpropamide
Glyburide
Patient Characteristics
Number of chronic health diagnoses (> 6)
Number of doses of medications per day (> 12)
Recent transfer from hospital
Advanced age (> 85)
Prior adverse drug reaction
Cancer
Depression
Low body weight or body mass index (< 22kg/m^2)
Six or more medications
Cognitive impairment including dementia
Decreased renal function (estimated creatinine clearance < 50ml/min)
Class of Medications
Anticonvulsants
Antiarrhythmics
Antipsychotics
Antidepressants
Sedative/hypnotics
Benzodiazepines
Histamine$_2$-antagonists
Nonsteroidal anti-inflammatory drugs
Anticholinergics
Angiotensin converting enzyme inhibitors
Diuretics
New prescription for antibiotic
Narcotic analgesic

Source: Fouts, M., Hanlon, J., Pieper, C., Perfetto, E., & Feinberg, J.: Identification of elderly nursing facility residents at high risk of drug-related problems. *Consult Pharm* 1997; 12[10]: 1103-11.

rize them. However, the PDPs have no financial incentive to provide these services, as for example, improving compliance with drug therapy will actually increase drug utilization and costs, which reduces their profitability. It is important, therefore, that an alternative mechanism exist to identify targeted beneficiaries and authorize the provision of MTM Services by a qualified health professional. The patient's primary care physician is a logical individual to identify and refer targeted beneficiaries for these services. Other individuals who may be able to identify these high-risk beneficiaries include Home Health nurses and admitting nurses at assisted living residences; pharmacists; social workers; and geriatric care managers and hospital discharge planners. Processes such as those being developed by Partners' Medication Management Model can be used as guidelines to establish and authorize pharmacist interventions for home health and other community-based programs.

DEFINING MEDICATION THERAPY MANAGEMENT SERVICES

What are MTM Services? In order to define MTM Services, it is important to first establish goals of providing such services. ASCP advocates that the goals must be to (see Table 2):

TABLE 2. ASCP Proposed Medication Management Service Goals

1. Ensure that Medicare beneficiaries are only taking medications that have a current and valid indication for use, reducing "polypharmacy."

2. Alert the prescriber when an individual has an apparent indication for drug therapy that is currently untreated.

3. Evaluate, and assist the prescriber, in monitoring whether the desired therapeutic outcomes are being achieved.

4. Evaluate the beneficiary for presence or high risk of adverse outcomes from medication use, including drug interactions, drug side effects and other adverse events such as falls, mental confusion, and delirium.

5. Monitor and encourage adherence to prescribed medications.

6. Simplify and reduce overall costs of the drug regimen.

7. Detailed review of medications in patients who are experiencing adverse outcomes, such as falls or urinary incontinence.

8. Design and implement medication management strategies to prevent the beneficiary from having to move to more "restrictive" levels of care.

1. *Ensure that Medicare beneficiaries are only taking medications that have a current and valid indication for use, reducing "polypharmacy."* Older adults frequently continue to take medications even after the medical problem is resolved. They may also receive similar medications for the same problem from more than one prescriber, resulting in duplicate drug therapy.
2. *Alert the prescriber when an individual has an apparent indication for drug therapy that is currently untreated.* Pneumococcal vaccine is an example of a drug product that is indicated for nearly all older adults, but is widely underused. Medications for depression and pain are also underutilized in the geriatric population.
3. *Evaluate, and assist the prescriber, in monitoring whether the desired therapeutic outcomes are being achieved.*
4. *Evaluate the beneficiary for presence or high risk of adverse outcomes from medication use, including drug interactions, drug side effects and other adverse events such as falls, mental confusion, and delirium.*
5. *Monitor and encourage adherence to prescribed medications.* Some ASCP members have identified that a large gap in medication management services for seniors today has to do with adherence. As an example, the Medication Education for Drug Safety or MEDS Program, in Raleigh, North Carolina, a community-based medication management program affiliated with a geriatric care management agency, noted that client non-adherence is one of the most common reasons for referral from physicians and social workers. Seniors benefit from in-home evaluation, education and then ongoing follow-up interventions such as pillbox and syringe fills. The service has successfully delayed and in some cases prevented nursing home placement, more costly than paying for syringe fills and pillbox fills and a quarterly evaluation.
6. *Simplify and reduce overall costs of the drug regimen.* MTM Services can reduce drug costs both for the payer and for the patient, by evaluating the overall drug regimen and exploring ways to achieve the same therapeutic objectives with lower cost alternatives. The pharmacist's broad knowledge of drug costs and PDP formulary and drug benefit design can be applied to work with high-cost patients to achieve these objectives. Some pharmacists have focused community-based practice on simplifying and streamlining medication regimens, thereby reducing medication costs for low-income seniors (Hogan, 2004).

7. *Detailed review of medications in patients who are experiencing adverse outcomes, such as falls or urinary incontinence.* Many medications can cause or contribute to a variety of geriatric syndromes or conditions. A pharmacist with geriatric expertise can evaluate the drug therapy of these individuals and recommend drug regimen changes to reduce these problems and improve functionality and quality of life for the older individual.

8. *Design and implement medication management strategies to prevent the beneficiary from having to move to more "restrictive" levels of care, such as helping the individual remain at home or in an assisted living setting instead of moving to a nursing home.* This may include special packaging provided by the pharmacy at the time of dispensing.

MTM Services may be provided by a pharmacist who may or may not be associated with the pharmacy that dispenses medication to the patient although some MTM Services could be associated with the dispensing of a drug product, and provided by the dispensing pharmacy. Services can be provided in a variety of community settings as described in Table 3.

The MTM Services provided by these pharmacists include the following:

- Comprehensive review of the patient drug regimen to identify, resolve, and prevent MRPs; this includes review of over-the-counter and herbal or alternative medicine products, along with prescription drugs.

TABLE 3. Pharmacist Settings for Medication Therapy Management Services

- A visit to the patient's home
- An office at the pharmacist's home or business setting
- Senior center or adult day service center
- Area Agency on Aging office
- Assisted living community
- A separate office within a community pharmacy setting
- Physician office or physician group practice

- Evaluation of outcomes of drug therapy (e.g., whether pain medications are providing adequate relief) or recommendations for achieving optimal outcomes of drug therapy (e.g., recommending dose or medication change to enhance pain management).
- Evaluation of possible adverse effects of drug therapy. In the elderly, medication side-effects are often misinterpreted and treated with new medications.
- Evaluation of patient compliance or adherence to drug therapy, and patient counseling or education to improve adherence to drug therapy.
- Collaboration with the prescriber(s) to provide feedback on drug therapy and assist in coordination of drug therapy.
- Development and implementation of a medication management plan, in collaboration with the caregiver and others, to prevent the patient from having to move to a higher level of care (such as a nursing home).

Forty states now permit collaborative drug therapy management agreements between physicians and pharmacists. Pharmacists are often able to adjust dosages of medication or order needed laboratory tests for patients as part of these protocol arrangements. The services provided by pharmacists through such agreements should also qualify for compensation as part of MTM Services for Medicare beneficiaries.

An excellent example of these agreements involves monitoring individuals who take warfarin, a medication used to prevent blood clots. Warfarin must be dosed carefully and monitored closely to successfully prevent blood clots without causing serious bleeding as a side effect. Pharmacists often conduct these activities as part of anticoagulation clinics. Studies of pharmacists serving in anticoagulation clinics have shown excellent outcomes of care from these arrangements (Ernst & Brandt, 2003; Dager et al., 2000; Witt & Humphries, 2003; Anderson, 2004; Tschol et al., 2003).

WHO MAY PROVIDE MEDICATION THERAPY MANAGEMENT SERVICES?

If targeted beneficiaries are defined broadly, then it would be necessary to have a liberal definition of who can provide these services; this is true because a broad definition would include some lower risk individuals who may be adequately served by less qualified health professionals.

Also, a broad definition would make so many Medicare beneficiaries eligible for the services that the supply of health professionals with expertise in geriatric drug therapy would not be adequate to provide services to all the eligible individuals.

A more focused definition of targeted beneficiaries would limit the MTM Services to truly high-risk individuals. In this case, it would be appropriate to limit provider status to individuals who are truly qualified to manage frail elderly individuals with complex needs. Pharmacists, physicians, and gerontological nurse practitioners with geriatric drug therapy expertise would be suitable medication therapy service providers.

CMS OVERSIGHT OF MTM SERVICES TO TARGETED BENEFICIARIES

How will CMS ensure that targeted beneficiaries actually receive the MTM Services to help achieve optimal outcomes from medication therapy? CMS regulations and oversight will be critical to establishing a "level playing field" among all the PDPs to ensure equal access to these services among Medicare beneficiaries.

Prescription Drug Plans could implement obstacles that would hinder beneficiaries from receiving MTM services. This may be done in three ways:

- Authorizing payment for these services using very stringent criteria that limit the number of eligible individuals (who can receive these services).
- Imposing stringent criteria for individuals who are authorized to provide services.
- Providing such a low level of payment that it is not economically feasible for qualified health professionals to provide these services.

CMS can address each of these issues in the regulations to implement the provision of MTM Services. In addition, CMS should implement a process to ensure that the regulations are followed. This could include having the PDPs provide a regular report on the provision of these services to targeted beneficiaries enrolled in their programs. The Quality Improvement Organizations (QIOs) could also be engaged in providing oversight of the PDPs, including the use of quality indicators to evaluate the services provided. As discussed above, many key questions remain unanswered in regards to the implementation of MTM Services that will begin in January 2006. Policy makers and administrators at CMS must look to the evidence-based programs such as the Home Health Medication Management Model as well as the numerous programs across the country that are addressing the medication needs of older adults at risk for medication-related problems. Key components of these programs can collectively lead to the answers that are critical if appropriate and cost effective MTM Services are to be delivered to our nation's most vulnerable citizens.

REFERENCES

Anderson, R.J. (2004). Cost analysis of a managed care decentralized outpatient pharmacy anticoagulation service. *Journal of Managed Care Pharmacy, 10*(2), 159-65.

Dager, W.E., Branch, J.M., King, J.H., White, R.H., Quan, R.S., Musallam, N.A. & Albertson, T.E. (2000). Optimization of inpatient warfarin therapy: Impact of daily consultation by a pharmacist-managed anticoagulation service. *Annals of Pharmacotherapy, 34*(5), 567-72.

Ernst, M.E., & Brandt, K.B. (2003). Evaluation of 4 years of clinical pharmacist anticoagulation case management in a rural, private physician office. *Journal of the American Pharmaceutical Association, 43*(5), 630-6.

Hogan, B. (September 2004). *The Pharmacist Who Says No to Drugs.* AARP Bulletin. Available at: http://www.aarp.org/bulletin/prescription/Articles/a2004-08-26-pharmacist. html. Accessed on November 2, 2004.

Meredith, S., Feldman, P., Frey, D., Giammarco, L., Hall, K., Arnold, K., Brown, N. J., & Ray, W.A. (2002). Improving medication use in home healthcare patients: A randomized controlled trial. *Journal of the American Geriatrics Society, 50,* 1484-1491.

Tschol, N., Lai, D.K.S., Tilley J.A., Wong, H., & Brown, G.R. (2003). Comparison of physician- and pharmacist-managed warfarin sodium treatment in open heart surgery patients. *Canadian Journal of Cardiology, 19*(12), 1413-7.

Upchurch, G.A., Menon, M.P., Levin, K.S., Catellier, D.J., & Conlisk, E.A. (2001). Prescription assistance for older adults with limited incomes: Client and program characteristics. *Journal of Pharmacy Technology, 17,* 6-12.

Witt, D.M., & Humphries, T.L. (2003). A retrospective evaluation of the management of excessive anticoagulation in an established clinical pharmacy anticoagulation service compared to traditional care. *Journal of Thrombosis & Thrombolysis, 15*(2), 113-8.

Polypharmacy and Possible Drug-Drug Interactions Among Diabetic Patients Receiving Home Health Care Services

Ibrahim A. Ibrahim, MD, MPH, PhD
Eunjeong Kang, PhD
Kathryn H. Dansky, RN, PhD

SUMMARY. *Objectives:* In this study, we examined the drug regimens of diabetic patients receiving home health care services to measure the prevalence of polypharmacy and to assess the likelihood of drug-drug interactions, a consequence of polypharmacy.

Design: The sample consisted of 139 diabetic patients who received home health care services from one home health agency in a large

Ibrahim A. Ibrahim is Director, Urology Outcomes Research, Beaumont Hospital, Urology Department. Eunjeong Kang is Research Associate, Korean Institute for Health and Social Affairs, Seoul, South Korea. Kathryn H. Dansky is Associate Professor, Department of Health Policy and Administration, The Pennsylvania State University.

Address correspondence to: Dr. Ibrahim A. Ibrahim, Beaumont Hospital, Director, Urology Outcomes Research, Urology Department, 3535 West 13 Mile Road, Suite 407A, Royal Oak, MI 48073-6769.

The authors would like to thank Larry S. Dansky, MD, of the Student Health Services at Pennsylvania State University for his helpful comments.

[Haworth co-indexing entry note]: "Polypharmacy and Possible Drug-Drug Interactions Among Diabetic Patients Receiving Home Health Care Services." Ibrahim, Ibrahim A., Eunjeong Kang, and Kathryn H. Dansky. Co-published simultaneously in *Home Health Care Services Quarterly* (The Haworth Press, Inc.) Vol. 24, No. 1/2, 2005, pp. 87-99; and: *Improving Medication Management in Home Care: Issues and Solutions* (ed: Dennee Frey) The Haworth Press, Inc., 2005, pp. 87-99. Single or multiple copies of this article are available for a fee from The Haworth Document Delivery Service [1-800-HAWORTH, 9:00 a.m. - 5:00 p.m. (EST). E-mail address: docdelivery@haworthpress.com].

mid-Atlantic city. The data were collected from March 1, 1998 to September 30, 1999. Information regarding medications was collected by the home health nurse during the initial home visit and was recorded on the medication sheet in the patient's clinical record. Any changes in medications were noted on the medication sheets.

Methods: We identified all systemic medications prescribed for 139 home health patients. To assess drug-drug interactions, we used Micromedex® formulary DRUG-REAX® System.

Outcomes: We calculated (1) the number of systemic medications taken, and (2) the number of possible severe, moderate, and mild drug-drug interactions.

Results: We found that the average number of medications taken was 8.9 (SD 3.4) prescribed medications per day. Our results show that 38.8% of the patients in the sample could potentially be subject to at least one severe drug-drug interaction. Nearly all of the patients (92.8%) were at risk for moderate drug-drug interactions, and 70.5% could have mild drug-drug interactions.

Conclusion: We conclude that polypharmacy is a concern for home health care patients with diabetes and the potential for drug-drug interactions is substantial. Our results indicate that the drug regimens of diabetic patients should be monitored systematically to avoid adverse events such as hospitalization. Family practitioners and home health care takers are in a unique position to identify polypharmacy and to modify drug regimens. *[Article copies available for a fee from The Haworth Document Delivery Service: 1-800-HAWORTH. E-mail address: <docdelivery@ haworthpress.com> Website: <http://www.HaworthPress.com> © 2005 by The Haworth Press, Inc. All rights reserved.]*

KEYWORDS. Polypharmacy, drug-drug interaction, diabetes, home health practitioners, elderly care, drug monitoring

INTRODUCTION

Polypharmacy is common among the elderly by virtue of the prevalence of chronic conditions in this population (Beyth and Shorr, 1999). For diabetic patients, polypharmacy is often inevitable given the potential for diabetes-related complications and other co-morbid conditions. Patients who are simultaneously taking many medications at the same time have higher chances of drug-drug interactions, drug-food interactions, and/or adverse drug reactions (Simmonson, 1984). Among these three negative consequences, drug-drug interaction (DDI) is the most serious and is the focus of this paper.

Drug interactions may lead to lower effectiveness of a treatment, physiological changes, or, sometimes lethal outcomes. Despite the importance of the issue, there has been little empirical research on DDI among diabetic patients (White and Campbell, 1995). This issue is a concern for family practitioners. As the primary care providers for most adult diabetics, they are in a unique position to identify polypharmacy, modify drug regimens and communicate information about pharmaceutical therapy among specialists and other health care providers.

There is no consensus on the definition of polypharmacy. In one study, polypharmacy was defined as a drug regimen including at least one unnecessary medication (Colley and Lucas, 1993). Another study defined it as "the long term simultaneous use of 2 or more drugs," with long term defined as > 240 days in a year (Veehof, Stewart, Haaijer-Juskamp, and Jong, 2000). Still another study defined polypharmacy as a drug regimen including more than five drugs (Fillit et al., 1999; Hanlon et al., 1997). Because possible drug-drug interactions increase exponentially with every drug added to the existing combination of drugs, we adopted the definition of polypharmacy as the use of five or more drugs simultaneously.

Polypharmacy is prevalent in the elderly, primarily because they have many co-morbid conditions. Previous research estimated that in U.S. nursing homes, the average number of drugs prescribed to residents was 7.2-8.1 (Broderick, 1997). Golden and his colleagues found that in homebound elderly, the average number of drugs taken was 5.3 ± 2.9 with a wide range of 0-22 (Golden et al., 1997). Similarly, in a large study of 6,178 home healthcare elderly population, it was found that the median number of medications taken was five with a sizable proportion of 19 percent of the patients taking nine or more medications (Meredith et al., 2001).

In the year 2000, there were 11 million people diagnosed with diabetes in the United States and this number is expected to grow much higher to 29 million by the year 2050. This is an increase of 165%, but the increase is predicted to be even higher (271% in women and 437% in men) among the elderly of 75 years and over (Boyle et al., 2001). The cost of care for diabetes was estimated at $98.2 billion in 1997 and the direct cost of nursing home care for diabetes in the same year was estimated to be $5,510 million (American Diabetes Association, 1998).

Diabetic patients are especially at high risk of polypharmacy because they are likely to have several diabetes-related complications such as ischemic heart disease, congestive heart failure, infections, peripheral vascular disease, renal disease, and amputations. Older individuals also have a higher chance of having other co-morbid conditions such as hypertension, peptic ulcer, rheumatoid arthritis, and cancer. The preceding discussion further supports examining possible medication problems among elderly diabetics.

This study aims at examining the prevalence of polypharmacy among a group of home healthcare elderly diabetic patients and to examine the possibility of drug-drug interactions between the prescribed medications to these patients. This will further add to the body of literature calling attention for this problem in general and among elderly in particular. It will also add credence to the possible threats of such a phenomenon to the quality of care delivered to this vulnerable group of patients.

METHODS

The original study sample consisted of diabetic patients who were discharged from the hospital with a referral to a home health agency in a large, mid-Atlantic city. These patients received skilled nursing visits either through telehomecare (using remote home visits via telemedicine using videophones connecting the visiting nurse to the homecare patients) or through traditional on site home visits. Data were collected from March 1998 through September 1999. Information regarding medications was collected by the home health nurse during the initial home visit and was recorded on medication sheets. Medication sheets were available for 139 out of 176 patients, thus the sample for this follow-up study is 139 patients.

Medication sheets were not available for 37 patients. Table 1 illustrates the comparisons of our sample and the excluded group in terms of demographic characteristics and disease status. Both groups showed a predominance of females and African Americans. Both groups showed a small proportion with education above high school and about three co-morbid conditions in addition to diabetes. Based on statistical tests of significance between the two groups, we concluded that the groups were equivalent except in age where the missing individuals were older and with somewhat lower diabetes severity.

The medication regimen of each patient was reviewed to identify prescribed medications. Medications considered for polypharmacy included only systemic drugs. Two groups of medications were not considered in assessing polypharmacy, namely, topical and over the

TABLE 1. Comparisons between our study sample and the excluded sample

	Study Sample (n = 139) n or Mean (% or SD)	Excluded Subjects (n = 37) n or Mean (% or SD)
Mean age**	73.6 (9.50)	78.0 (6.76)
Gender		
Male	39 (28.7%)	9 (20.0%)
Female	97 (71.3%)	27 (80.0%)
Race		
Black, non-Hispanic	90 (67.2%)	24 (75.0%)
White, non-Hispanic	44 (32.8%)	6 (25.0%)
Mean years of education	10.5 (2.8)	10.9 (3.4)
Mean number of co-morbidities	3.0	3.1
Mean diabetes severity*	2.4	2.0

* $p < .05$ ** $p < .01$

counter medications. Topical and ophthalmic drugs were excluded, because they have an effect mainly on the targeted local area while over-the-counter medications were not considered in this study because of the difficulty to document and the universality of access to them by all patients. Furthermore, different types of insulin were considered as one drug and collapsed into one insulin category.

We used a Micromedex® drug-drug interaction system, DRUG-REAX,® to check possible drug-drug interactions. This system was made available to the authors free of charge for the purpose of this study. Micromedex drug interaction database was examined independently and found to be strongly supportable for use in clinical practice (Kupferberg and Hartel, 2004; Gaddis, Holt, and Woods, 2002; Langdorf et al., 2000). Each drug interaction is classified into one of three-levels of severity categories: severe, moderate, and mild. "Severe" interactions mean that death and/or life-threatening injuries have been reported in similar drug combinations. "Moderate" interactions were found to be associated with drugs for which serious, but non-lethal and non-life-threatening injuries have been reported. "Mild" interactions occur when clinically insignificant effects and neutral or even favorable effects have been reported for these interactions. The severity category represents the severity of the potential interaction if it occurs and does not assess the likelihood that the interaction may occur. Since only severe and moderate interactions may be related to adverse drug events and hospitalizations, our analysis considered only these two categories of interactions as undesirable.

For the measurement of co-morbidity, we used two variables: one for diabetes-related co-morbid conditions and one for other co-morbid conditions that are not necessarily diabetes-related. The number of co-morbidities was measured as a continuous variable with a range from 0 to 4. Severity of diabetes was assessed for each patient on admission to home health care services. The general condition severity variables were measured with Likert scales that are part of the Outcome and Assessment Information Set "OASIS" data set, a standardized data collection instrument mandated by the Health Care Financing Administration for all Medicare-certified home health agencies.

We carried out a bi-variate correlation analysis linking the disease specific patient characteristics such as number of co-morbidities, number of complications, and degree of diabetes severity; and the number of medications taken by these diabetic patients. This type of analysis considers the cross product of deviations and co-variances for each pair of variables. The resulting Pearson correlation coefficient is reported.

RESULTS

The number and types of medications were examined and the means +/− standard deviation were reported. Our study sample has a disproportionately large number of black and other minority patients (67%), and three times as many females as males due to the prevailing demographics in the study region. The average age was 74. The average diabetes severity score was 2.4 (range of 1-4). The diabetes severity score of "2" means that symptoms were controlled with difficulty, while "3" means that symptoms were poorly controlled with frequent treatment adjustments. The average number of co-morbidities was 3 (Table 1).

The average number of all systemic medications prescribed to these diabetic patients was 8.9 (SD = 3.4) with the range between 2 and 19 medications. Cardiovascular, anti-inflammatory and analgesic, and antidiabetic drugs were prescribed most frequently for the patients in this sample (2.6/day, 1.2/day, 1.1/day, respectively). We found that 88% of the patients were subjects for polypharmacy, i.e., they were taking more than 5 medications simultaneously. Our results show that 38.8% of the patients in the sample could potentially be subject to at least one severe drug-drug interaction (DDI). Nearly all the patients (92.8%) could potentially have moderate DDI and 70.5% could have mild DDI. The average number of potential drug-drug interactions per patient was 8.6 ($\pm$ 7.3), with the possibility of 0.7 ($\pm$ 1.1) severe interactions, 5.7 ($\pm$ 4.9) moderate interactions, and 2.3 ($\pm$ 3.1) mild interactions. In Table 2, we provide examples of the drug interactions that were identified as being most likely to result in severe DDI. The most frequent severe drug-drug interactions were the combinations of diuretics with non-steroid anti-inflammatory drugs (39.8%), and diuretics with digoxin (18.3%). However, it should be mentioned that a combination like furosemide with digoxin, although commonly and appropriately used together, should be carefully monitored and treated for diuretic-induced hypokalemia or hypomagnesemia which may put patients using digoxin at risk for arrhythmias. Fourteen patients (15.1%) were prescribed Coumadin and NSAID simultaneously. Although they act synergistically and often

TABLE 2. Examples of severe drug-drug interactions

	Example	Frequency (%)
Diuretic-NSAID	Furosemide-aspirin	37 (39.8)
Diuretic-antihypertensive	Furosemide-digoxin and bumetanide-digoxin*	17 (18.3)
Anticoagulant-NSAID	Coumadin-aspirin	14 (15.1)
Cardiac agent-antihypertensive	Verapamil-digoxin, atenolol-verapamil	8 (8.6)
CNS agent-CNS agent	Fluoxetine-imipramin, haloperidol-sinemet, elavil-fluoxetine	3 (3.2)
CNS agent-analgesic	Carbamazepine-tramadol, norpramin-tramadol	2 (2.1)
Other	Captopril-allopurinol, vasotec-allopurinol, coumadin-tamoxifen, coumadin-ampicillin, coumadin-synthroid, coumadin-amiodarone, coumadin-cyclosporin, cyclosporin-pravachol	12 (12.9)
Total		93 (100.0)

* Although diuretics and digitalis glycosides are frequently and appropriately used together, there is a potential for diuretics like furosemide to induce hypokalemia and hypomagnesemia which may put the patient on digoxin at risk of arrhythmias. Therefore, potassium and magnesium levels should be followed closely to allow early identification and treatment of hypokalemia and hypomagnesemia.

prescribed for prevention of further stroke or fibrillation (Christian, Lapane, and Toppa, 2003), these two medications were not recommended for routine use together in the elderly (Dhond, Michelena, and Ezekowitz, 2003 and Reikvam, Madsen, and Landmark, 2003). A combination of Verapamil and digoxin or atenolol and verapamil were noted in 8 patients. Again, although extreme reactions were reported using these combinations (Sakurai et al., 2000), for the most part there were no adverse reactions in the field with prevalent use in essential hypertension.

Table 3 identifies factors correlated with the number of medications taken by patients in this sample. Age and diabetes severity were significantly correlated to the number of medications prescribed but in different directions. Surprisingly, age was negatively associated with polypharmacy. This finding was unexpected because older diabetic patients typically have more co-morbid conditions and often a more severe form of the disease. As one would expect, the degree of diabetes severity was positively associated with the number of medications prescribed. The number of co-morbidities was not significantly correlated with the number of medications prescribed.

DISCUSSION

Our results indicate that diabetic patients receiving home health services were prescribed more medications (mean = 8.9, SD = 3.38) than their nursing home or homebound elderly counterparts reported in the literature. Previous studies found that the average number of medica-

TABLE 3. Factors correlated with the number of medications taken by diabetic patients

	Coefficients* (p value)
Age**	−0.186 (p = 0.014)
Co-morbidity	0.007 (p = 0.936)
Diabetes co-morbidity	−0.084 (p = 0.308)
Diabetes severity**	0.208 (p = 0.013)

* These are Pearson correlation coefficients and their associated p value
**p < .05

tions was 7.2-8.1 for nursing home residents (Broderic, 1997) and 5.3 (SD = 2.9) for homebound elderly (Golden et al., 1997). Our results suggest that diabetic patients use more medications than the average elderly, confirming our earlier suspicion that diabetic patients may be at higher risk of polypharmacy.

A high proportion of patients (38.8%) were at risk for severe DDI. Severe drug interactions can cause life-threatening events. For example, aspirin may increase the risk of bleeding when a patient takes warfarin by inhibiting platelet aggregation and inducing gastrointestinal bleeding. These common complications and co-morbid conditions raise concerns regarding the concurrent use of ß-blockers, diuretics, and non-steroid anti-inflammatory drug (NSAIDs).

However, we have few caveats here. First, not all drug-drug interactions flagged out by drug interaction software, actually result in adverse drug events. Each medication has its own pharmacokinetics, i.e., the patterns of absorption, distribution, and excretion in the body. Even if several medications are taken at the same time, not all the medications are absorbed at the same time, site or rate. Second, the occurrence of DDI also depends on organ functioning. While absorption may take place in the gastrointestinal tract, detoxification occurs in the liver and excretion takes place in the kidneys. A disease process that affects any of these organs may result in delayed absorption, distribution, or excretion. Therefore, the occurrence of DDI depends on the patient's functional status. Of course, if medications are taken at different times, the chance of drug interactions may decrease.

We found that the oldest old do not take as many diabetic medications as younger elderly. This finding was echoed in the literature. For example, Glynn and colleagues found that diabetic medication use decreased as age increased (Glynn et al., 1999). They conjectured that this was partly because physicians do not expect treatment effects of medications in the oldest old as much as in other younger elderly. They also suggested that this age group had more diabetic complications and therefore patients needed other medications for controlling these complications rather than controlling blood glucose itself. It has also been found that the oldest-old were at a higher risk for drug-associated hypoglycemia (Shorr, Ray, Daugherty, and Griffith, 1997). This may be explained by the fact that their kidney and liver functions are so weak that anti-diabetic drugs cannot be excreted at their normal excretion rates. Instead these drugs stay in the circulation longer than they do in younger people. This indicates the need for more research into why the oldest-old use fewer diabetic medications.

According to our findings, NSAIDs and diuretics are most frequently involved in possible DDI with anti-diabetic drugs. Even though the new generations of sulfonylurea (Glipizide, Glyburide) are relatively less likely to interact with protein-binding drugs like NSAIDs, there is a need to evaluate adverse reactions closely when sulfonylurea therapy is initiated or discontinued (Sone, Takahashi, and Yamada, 2001). Diuretics, especially thiazide diuretics, have been identified as interacting agents with anti-diabetic drugs (Wolff and Lindeman, 1966; Amery et al., 1978; Cowley and Elkeles, 1978; Harrower, 2000). Despite this, they are still widely used with anti-diabetic drugs. Thiazide diuretics also decrease the anti-diabetic effect of anti-diabetic drugs; therefore careful monitoring when prescribing and administering these drugs is indicated. However, this presents a case for reviewing interactions reported by software checking DDI and use more evidence-based literature than traditionally known theoretically incompatible drug combinations.

CONCLUSION

Polypharmacy is prevalent among the elderly with diabetes in home health care. This may be inevitable considering complications of diabetes and other co-morbid conditions among the elderly. Polypharmacy, as a result, raises many concerns about drug-drug interactions and possible negative consequences such as adverse drug events and hospitalizations. In this study of diabetic elderly receiving home health care services, we found that 88% of the patients experienced polypharmacy. We also found that 38.8% of these elderly persons could have been subject to severe drug-drug interactions.

For effective and safe care of the diabetic elderly, careful management of medications is critical. One of the most effective strategies is, of course, to simplify the drug regimen. This can be accomplished by eliminating pharmacological duplication, decreasing the frequency of medication administration, and reducing the dose itself whenever possible (Colley and Lucas, 1993; Cohen, 2000). Monitoring drug regimens is another method of reducing the risk involved in polypharmacy by enhancing the early detection of possible drug-related problems. There is a need for a wide use of pharmacy consultation model similar to the one reported by Brown et al. to focus on consensus-based identification and resolution of the most prevalent and serious medication problems in the home health care setting (Brown et al., 1998).

Community pharmacies and home health professionals may be the link that can flag out possible drug-drug interactions and subsequently inform the health care provider who prescribed the medications. Case managers also can monitor patients' medication use and detect possible drug-drug interactions.

Primary care physicians and pharmacists should give patients relevant information about their drug regimen so that patients know which drugs they are taking. Any over-the-counter (OTC) medications taken by the patient should also be included in the medical record. Periodically, patients should bring in all medications, particularly those prescribed by different providers, to ensure that their current family practitioner in charge has accurate information on the drug regimen. With this information in hand, physicians can discuss the potential for drug-drug interactions with their patients, and together they can determine the most appropriate medication management plan.

Future polypharmacy research should focus on management of complex medication regimens and strategies to reduce drug-drug interactions. How to involve pharmacists and other health care providers is critical for improving home health patient outcomes. There is also a need for prospective studies to monitor actual occurrence of DDI and compare their incidence to potential reported by DDI detection software. This study is more of a theoretical exercise to draw attention to the problem but at the same time it needs further validation in the field.

Limitations

Several limitations have to be noted here. Our study, being based on a convenience sample, has a large majority of black and other minorities that do not project to the entire U.S. population. Furthermore, the DDI reported here represent the potential interactions rather than interactions that already took place. Finally, although the severity scales in the OASIS data set have been validated (Shaugnessy et al., 1993), they are still based on clinical judgment, and may be subjective and therefore prone to measurement errors.

Key Points for Practitioners

- The average number of medications taken by diabetic elderly was 8.9 (± 3.4).
- Our results show that 38.8% of the patients in the sample could potentially be subject to at least one severe drug-drug interaction.
- Nearly all the patients (92.8%) could potentially have moderate drug-drug interactions.

REFERENCES

American Diabetes Association. (1998). Economic consequences of diabetes mellitus in the United States in 1997. *Diabetes Care, 21*, 296-309.

Amery, A. et al. (1978). Glucose intolerance during diuretic therapy. *Lancet, 1*, 681.

Beyth, R.J., & Shorr, R.I. (1999). Epidemiology of adverse drug reactions in the elderly by drug category. *Drugs Aging, 14*(3), 231-239.

Boyle, J.P., Honeycutt, A.A., Venkat Narayan, K.M., Hoerger, T.J., Geiss, L.S., Chen, H., & Thompson, T.J. (2001). Projection of Diabetes Burden Through 2050: Impact of Changing Demography and Disease Prevalence in the United States. *Diabetes Care, 24*(11), 1936-1940.

Broderick, E. (1997). Prescribing patterns for nursing home residents in the U.S. The reality and the vision. *Drugs & Aging, 11*(4), 255-260.

Brown, N.J., Griffin, M.R., Ray, W.A., Meredith, S., Beers, M.H., Marren, J., Robles, M., Stergachis, A., Wood, A.J., and Avorn, J. (1998). A Model for Improving Medication Use in Home Health Care Patients. *Journal of the American Pharmaceutical Association, 38*, 696-702.

Christian, J.B., Lapane, K.L., & Toppa, R.S. (2003). Racial disparities in receipt of secondary stroke prevention agents among U.S. nursing home residents. *Stroke, 34*(11), 2693- 2697.

Cohen, J.S. Avoiding adverse reactions. (2000). Effective lower-dose drug therapies for older patients. *Geriatrics, 55*(2), 54-64.

Colley, C.A., & Lucas, L.M. (1993). Polypharmacy: The cure becomes the disease. *Journal of General Internal Medicine, 8*(5), 278-83.

Cowley, A.J., & Elkeles, R.S. (1978). Diabetes and therapy with potent diuretics. *Lancet, 1*, 154.

de Leeuw, P.W., Notter, T., & Zilles, P. (1997). Comparison of different fixed antihypertensive combination drugs: A double blind, placebo-controlled parallel group study. *Journal of Hypertension, 15*, 87-91.

Dhond, A.J., Michelena, H.I., & Ezekowitz, M.D. (2003). Anticoagulation in the elderly. *Americcan Journal of Geriatric Cardiology, 12*(4), 243-250.

Fillit, H.M., Futterman, R., Orland, B.I., Chim, T., Susnow, L., Picariello, G.P., Scheye, E.C., Spoeri, R.K., Roglieri, J.L., & Warburton, S.W. (1999). Polypharmacy management in Medicare managed care: Changes in prescribing by primary care physicians resulting from a program promoting medication reviews. *Americna Journal of Managed Care, 5*(5), 587-94.

Gaddis, G.M., Holt, T.R., & Woods, M. (2002). Drug interactions in at-risk emergency department patients. *Academy of Emergency Medicine, 9*(11),1162-7.

Glynn, R.J., Monane, M., Gurwitz, J.H., Choodnovskiy, I., and Avorn, J. (1999). Aging, Comorbidity, and Reduced Rates of Drug Treatment for Diabetes Mellitus. *Journal of Clinical Epidemiology, 52*(8), 781-790.

Golden, A.G., Preston, R.A., Barnett, S.D., Llorente, M., Hamdan, K., & Silverman, M.A. (1997). Inappropriate medication prescribing in homebound older adult. *Journal of the American Geriatrics Society, 47*(8), 948-953.

Hanlon, J.T., Schmader, K.E., Koronkowski, M.J., Weinberger, M., Landsman, P.B., Samsa, G.P., & Lewis, I.K. (1997). Adverse drug events in high risk older outpatients. *Journal of American Geriatric Society, 45*(8), 945-8.

Harrower, A.D. (2000). Comparative tolerability of sulphonylureas in diabetes mellitus. *Drug Safety, 22*(4), 313-20.

Kupferberg, N., & Jones Hartel, L. (2004). Evaluation of five full-text drug databases by pharmacy students, faculty, and librarians: Do the groups agree? *Journal of Medical Library Association, 92*(1), 66-71.

Langdorf, M.I., Fox, J.C., Marwah, R.S., Montague, B.J., & Hart, M.M. (2000). Physician versus computer knowledge of potential drug interactions in the emergency department. *Acad Emerg Med., 7*(11), 1321-9.

Meredith, S., Feldman, P.H., Frey, D., Hall, K., Arnold, K., Brown, N.J., & Ray, W.A. (2001). Possible medication errors in home healthcare patients. *Journal of American Geriatric Society, 49*(6), 719-24.

Reikvam, A., Madsen, S., & Landmark, K. (2003). [Secondary prevention after acute myocardial infarction: Aspirin, warfarin or both?]. *Tidsskr Nor Laegeforen, 123*(13-14), 1838-40.

Sakurai, H., Kei, M., Matsubara, K., Yokouchi, K., Hattori, K., Ichihashi, R., Hirakawa, Y., Tsukamoto, H., & Saburi, Y. (2000). Cardiogenic shock triggered by verapamil and atenolol: A case report of therapeutic experience with intravenous calcium. *Japan Circ Journal, 64*(11), 893-6.

Shaughnessy, P.W., Crisler, K.S., & Schlenker, R.E. (1993). *Medicare OASIS: Standardized Outcome and Assessment Information Set for Home Health Care.* Center for Health Service and Policy Research, Denver, Colorado.

Shorr, R.I., Ray, W.A., Daugherty, J.R., & Griffin, M.R. (1997). Incidence and risk factors for serious hypoglycemia in older persons using insulin or sulfonylureas. *Archives of Internal Medicine, 157*(15), 1681-6.

Simonson, W. (1984). *Medications & The Elderly: A Guide for Promoting Proper Use.* An Aspen Publication.

Sone, H., Takahashi, A., & Yamada, N. (2001). Ibuprofen-related hypoglycemia in a patient receiving sulfonylurea. *Annals Internal Medicine, 134*(4), 344.

Veehof, L., Stewart, R., Haaijer-Juskamp, F., & Jong, B.M. (2000). The development of polypharmacy. A longitudinal study. *Family Practice, 17*(3), 261-267.

White, J.R. Jr., & Campbell, R.K. (1995). Drug/Drug and drug/disease interactions and diabetes. *Diabetes Educ, 21*(4), 283-286.

Wolff, F.W., & Lindeman, R.D. (1966). Effects of treatment in hypertension: Results of a controlled study. *Journal of Chronic Diseases, 19*, 227.

Opportunities for Improving Post-Hospital Home Medication Management Among Older Adults

Janice B. Foust, PhD, RN
Mary D. Naylor, PhD, RN, FAAN
Peter A. Boling, MD
Kimberly A. Cappuzzo, PharmD, MS

SUMMARY. Effective post-hospital home medication management among older adults is a convoluted, error-prone process. Older adults, whose complex medication regimens are often changed at hospital discharge, are susceptible to medication-related problems (e.g., Adverse Drug Events or ADEs) as they resume responsibility for managing their

---

Janice B. Foust is affiliated with the John A. Hartford Foundation, Building Academic Geriatric Nursing Capacity Scholar Program, University of Pennsylvania School of Nursing, and is Assistant Professor of Nursing, University of New Hampshire, Department of Nursing. Mary D. Naylor is affiliated with the University of Pennsylvania, School of Nursing. Peter A. Boling is affiliated with the Virginia Commonwealth University Health System, Division of Internal Medicine/General Internal Medicine/Primary Care. Kimberly A. Cappuzzo is affiliated with the Virginia Commonwealth University, Department of Pharmacy.

Address correspondence to: Dr. Janice B. Foust, University of New Hampshire, Department of Nursing, 251 Hewitt Hall, Durham, NH 03824 (E-mail: janice.foust@unh.edu).

The John A. Hartford Foundation, Building Academic Geriatric Nursing Capacity Program, is gratefully acknowledged for their support.

[Haworth co-indexing entry note]: "Opportunities for Improving Post-Hospital Home Medication Management Among Older Adults." Foust, Janice B. et al. Co-published simultaneously in *Home Health Care Services Quarterly* (The Haworth Press, Inc.) Vol. 24, No. 1/2, 2005, pp. 101-122; and: *Improving Medication Management in Home Care: Issues and Solutions* (ed: Dennee Frey) The Haworth Press, Inc., 2005, pp. 101-122. Single or multiple copies of this article are available for a fee from The Haworth Document Delivery Service [1-800-HAWORTH, 9:00 a.m. - 5:00 p.m. (EST). E-mail address: docdelivery@haworthpress.com].

medications at home. Human error theory frames the discussion of multi-faceted, interacting factors including care system functions, like discharge medication teaching that contribute to post-hospital ADEs. The taxonomy and causes of post-hospital ADEs and related risk factors are reviewed, as we describe in high-risk older adults a population that may benefit from targeted interventions. Potential solutions and future research possibilities highlight the importance of interdisciplinary teams, involvement of clinical pharmacists, use of transitional care models, and improved use of informational technologies. *[Article copies available for a fee from The Haworth Document Delivery Service: 1-800-HAWORTH. E-mail address: <docdelivery@haworthpress.com> Website: <http://www.HaworthPress. com> © 2005 by The Haworth Press, Inc. All rights reserved.]*

KEYWORDS. Older adults, medication management, medication errors, post-hospital, hospital discharge, human error theory, home care

INTRODUCTION

Effective post-hospital home medication management for older adults is laden with challenges. It requires consideration of elders' unique clinical needs and socioeconomic circumstances plus communication among numerous individuals across multiple sites. Prescriptions are commonly written in a hospital, handed to older adults or their families, reviewed with them before discharge, filled at a local pharmacy, and finally administered at home with or without professional supervision. Frequently, the discharge medications differ somewhat from those the patient took previously. The purpose of this paper is to describe post-hospital home medication problems faced by older adults within a context of human error theory (Reason, 1990; Reason, 1995). Post-hospital home medication management is defined, for the intent of this paper, as the interdisciplinary work of preparing and assisting patients to safely and accurately manage their medications at home after they leave the hospital. Potential solutions and considerations for future research will also be discussed.

In recent decades, the explosion of potent new pharmaceutical agents has greatly complicated medication management. Moreover, health care has become more fragmented with the evolution of setting-specific specialists: office-based primary care providers and sub-specialty medical consultants. Cost pressures have accelerated the pace of movement through the system, further compounding matters, and information sharing during transitions to post-hospital care can be inadequate, incomplete or inconsistent.

Medical errors is an appropriate framework for examining problems related to medication management at the time of transitions. The Institute of Medicine's (IOM) report "To Err is Human" has focused the public's attention on the problem of medical errors (Kohn, Corrigan, & Donaldson, 2000). Among those hospitalized, older adults experience more medical injuries (e.g., adverse drug events, falls) than younger patients (Brennan et al., 1991; Creditor, 1993; Rothschild, Bates, & Leape, 2000) and drug complications may be the most common medical injury (Leape et al., 1991). Older adults are at greater risk because of individual and age-related declines in physiological reserves, functional limitations, greater co-morbid disease burden, and sometimes, inappropriate geriatric care (Gurwitz & Avorn, 1991; Rothschild et al., 2000). For example, nearly all hospitalized frail older adults (91.9%) have at least one inappropriate medication, which reflect these geriatric issues, e.g., improper dosage, co-morbidity (Hanlon et al., 2004). Accurate prescribing for older adults is even more difficult because the elderly are not well represented in research trials, which further hinders the quality of evidence guiding pharmaceutical decisions (Gurwitz & Rochon, 2002).

The transition from hospital to home is a time of particularly high risk for errors. Yet, while numerous studies have focused on medication errors, scientific evidence related to errors occurring during the transition of older adults from hospital to home is less extensive. Most medication error research has been conducted in single institutions, and does not explore coordination of care among sites. Still, a few recent studies have uncovered serious post-hospital quality problems, and a majority of these have involved medications (Forster, Murff, Peterson, Gandhi, & Bates, 2003; Forster et al., 2004).

Discharge planning and hospital discharge activities are among the first steps to safe post-hospital care and a critical juncture where the priority areas of care coordination, self-care management and medication management coalesce (Adams & Corrigan, 2003). The American Geriatrics Society and others have stressed the need to identify system failures and correct gaps in the continuity of care to enhance quality of care and promote patient safety for older adults (Cook, Render, & Woods, 2000; Coleman, 2003; Tsilimingras, Rosen, & Berlowitz, 2003). Post-hospital home medication management is an area that deserves such attention.

MEDICATION SAFETY TERMINOLOGY

Many terms can be used in studies of medication safety. Medication errors are defined as problems occurring at any step in the process from ordering to administering a drug, regardless of patient response (Bates, Boyle, Vander Vliet, Schneider, & Leape, 1995). Adverse Drug Events (ADEs) are defined as situations when injury occurred as a result of an intervention related to a drug, which were deemed preventable if they were avoidable by current means (Bates et al., 1995). These terms will be used in this paper.

THEORETICAL FRAMEWORK: HUMAN ERROR THEORY

The IOM has suggested human error theory (Reason, 1990) as an approach to analyze failures in the healthcare system and create safer practices (Kohn et al., 2000). Human error theory emphasizes the links among errors, human fallibility, imperfect technology and the effects of organizational policies and immediate work environments (Reason, 1990; Reason, 1995). Errors are broadly classified as failures in planning (i.e., mistakes) or execution of the plan (i.e., slips and lapses) (Reason, 1995). These can occur at various phases of care such as establishing a diagnosis, designing and delivering treatment, or in communication among providers (Leape, 1994). Human error theory has been used to study ADEs in hospitals (Leape et al., 1995) and adapted for use in analyzing clinical risk (Vincent, Taylor-Adams, & Stanhope, 1998; Vincent et al., 2000). An advantage of the human error framework is its explicit connection of failures to individuals working in the context of specific local and organizational situations. Reason (1995) summarized conditions contributing to errors such as high workloads, inexperience, inadequate supervision, stressful environments and individuals' mental states (e.g., fatigue). Other factors influencing safe clinical practice include regulations, financial incentives, staffing levels, team communication, individual staff knowledge and abilities, ambiguous procedures, cognitive errors (e.g., omissions), inadequate information and patient characteristics, such as acuity, language or motivation (Bogner, 1994; Vincent et al., 1998). Human error theory similarly applies to the situations surrounding older adults' safe post-hospital home medication management.

CHALLENGES OF POST-HOSPITAL HOME MEDICATION MANAGEMENT

Post-hospital home medication management begins with discharge planning that is later implemented on the day of discharge when patients receive their prescriptions and instructions to help them resume continuing responsibility for their medications. Most studies of post-hospital care have followed patients between two weeks to three months after hospital discharge (Naylor et al., 1994; Gray, Mahoney, & Blough, 1999; Gray, Mahoney, & Blough, 2001; Forster et al., 2003; Forster et al., 2004; Smigelski, Hungate, & Boling, 2004). Other studies extended the time and followed patients from 6 months to a year after hospital discharge (Naylor et al., 1999; Naylor et al., 2004).

Errors in post-hospital home medication management can be organized as active or latent failures and will be presented in this paper (see Table 1). Incorrect prescriptions and medication discrepancies are more obvious errors, or active failures, because they can have more immediate effects (Reason, 1995). In contrast, inadequate discharge teaching, inattention to medication-related risk factors when choosing and dosing medications, and poor coordination of care may be considered latent failures because their effects, such as non-adherence or hospital admission, are more complex and delayed (Reason, 1995).

TABLE 1. Failures of Post-Hospital Home Medication Management

Definitions*	Examples
Active failures: Unsafe acts occurring at the point of patient contact that can have more immediate negative effects.	• Discharge prescription problems • Medication discrepancies
Latent failures: Errors stemming from organizational decisions that affect local work conditions and can go unnoticed until, through a series of events, a problem occurs much later.	• Abrupt shift in responsibility for medication management to older adults • Inattention to medication related risk factors • Flawed discharge medication teaching • Poor coordination and/or communication of medication changes at hospital discharge • Separate patient information records

* (Reason, 1995)

Post-Hospital Adverse Drug Events

In the month following hospital discharge, ADEs were the most frequent type of medical injury (66-72%) (Forster et al., 2003; Forster et al., 2004) and occurred in 20.3% of older adults receiving home care (Gray et al., 1999). Medication changes are frequent among patients discharged from hospitals. A majority of home care patients received at least one or two new prescriptions (53.3%) and some had three or more new medications (26.7%) at hospital discharge (Gray et al., 1999). Although a different population, hospitalized older adults returning to nursing homes experienced ADEs that were most often related to drugs stopped in the hospital and associated with comorbidity (Boockvar et al., 2004). Importantly, this study revealed a delay between drug changes and the onset of ADEs that typically spanned 14 days and incurred a 4.4% risk of an ADE with each medication change (Boockvar et al., 2004). Collectively, these studies illustrate the delayed and adverse impact of medication changes made in hospitals that can be potentially difficult for providers to anticipate or detect in other sites without adequate communication. Reason (1990) mentions feedback delay as a human error factor that can affect problem solving and diminish performance. Feedback is essential to refining practice skills and when it is absent ineffective care can continue unnoticed. Unfortunately, there are few, if any, post-hospital feedback mechanisms in place.

The consequences of ADEs can be serious, including hospitalization and death. Preventable drug-related hospitalizations have resulted from inappropriate dosing, development of abnormal laboratory findings, inadequate monitoring, patient non-adherence and drug interactions (McDonnell & Jacobs, 2002). Drug-drug interactions represented 60.6% of the ADEs on admission (Doucet et al., 2002) and specific interactions (e.g., potassium-sparing diuretics and angiotensin converting enzyme inhibitors) were a source of preventable hospital admissions (2.3-7.8%) (Juurlink, Mamdani, Kopp, Laupacis, & Redelmeier, 2003). A note of caution is due: two of these studies (Doucet et al., 2002; Juurlink et al., 2003) were conducted in France and Canada and may not reflect the situation in the United States.

We can now turn to research that has elucidated some of the contributing mechanisms to these serious problems.

Discharge Prescription Problems

Studies have revealed discharge prescription error rates of 5.8-18% (Chan, Maxwell, Koger, Gamboa, & Brewer, 1990; Schumock, Guenette,

Keys, & Hutchinson, 1994). Types of active errors included duplicate, omitted or incomplete prescriptions and incorrect directions or doses (Chan et al., 1990; Schumock et al., 1994; Chantelois & Suzuki, 2003). An omitted discharge prescription is an especially obscure and potentially dangerous error, and it may be difficult to accurately identify. In some cases, the drugs are intentionally omitted from the post-hospital regimen, while in others older adults wrongly assume that the omitted medication is no longer needed. Factors contributing to omissions when discharging patients include performing isolated and repetitive work (e.g., prescriptions, discharge summaries, discharge instructions) in a hurry immediately before a patient leaves the hospital (Reason, 2002). Other discharge prescription problems, such as improper dosing, may be due to distractions or knowledge-based errors (Reason, 1990) when providers fail to address the patient's specific situation (e.g., poor renal function). Reconciling a patient's medication regimens from the period prior to admission, during the hospital stay, and at discharge could lessen some of these prescribing problems and verify changes, but this can be time consuming (Rozich & Resar, 2001).

Medication Discrepancies

Medication discrepancies are already evident during outpatient care of older adults (Beers, Sliwkowski, & Brooks, 1992; Bedell et al., 2000). Patients took medications not recorded in their clinic charts (51-64%); omitted a recorded medication (29-50%); or took medication differently than recorded (20-73%) (Beers et al., 1992; Bedell et al., 2000). Discrepancies were associated with increasing patient age and number of recorded medications among outpatients and post-hospital home care patients (Bedell et al., 2000; Lewis, Pavlis, Chen, & Fields, 2004). Elderly home care patients also adjusted their medications and were found to take less than the intended amount of prescribed medications and more "as needed" medications than listed (Hsia Der, Rubenstein, & Choy, 1997).

At hospital discharge, we add another group of new providers, plus multiple hand-offs: from hospital to home health agency, from hospital pharmacy to community pharmacy, and from hospital physicians to office providers. The interface between hospital-based and post-hospital providers may employ written referrals, discharge summaries, letters, phone calls, or in too many cases no formal communication of any kind. The timelines and accuracy of these records are inconsistent. Accordingly, a recent study found 42% of recently discharged patients had a medication discrepancy when comparing hospital discharge plans and first outpatient visit records (Moore, Wisnivesky, Williams, & McGinn, 2003). In addition to patient choice, sources of medication discrepancies include fragmented communication among professionals (Vincent et al., 1998) that is aggravated by a system that requires each setting (e.g., hospitals, clinics) to maintain and protect patient records and assure privacy.

Flawed Discharge Medication Teaching

The day of hospital discharge is a vitally important yet potentially unsafe time to prepare older adults to manage their medications at home. For professionals, there are several key steps that include: choosing the correct medication, writing an accurate prescription, providing the patient with the prescription, determining whether the patient will be able to obtain the prescribed medication in a timely manner, reviewing prescriptions with patients and families, making sure that changes from previous regimens are clear, noting major potential adverse reactions, and communicating the new regimen accurately to professional post-hospital care providers who will assume responsibility for the patient's ongoing care.

From the older adult's perspective, there is an abrupt shift in the responsibility for medication management. While hospitalized, older adults have little control over their medications. Yet, they are expected to assume immediate and often complete responsibility at discharge. Therefore, discharge medication teaching is an important process that passes the "baton of responsibility" from professionals to patients. Additionally, patients and families, who may be stressed or exhausted after the hospitalization, must implement medication regimens at home within their available resources and abilities. This situation is open to human error at many levels.

Discharge medication teaching is essential to prepare older adults to manage their medications at home. Physicians, nurses and pharmacists whose roles vary with hospital policies, local and individual practice patterns, and available resources should share this activity. One study revealed that nurses provided discharge medication teaching in a variety of ways, including informal preparation throughout the hospitalization and more formal instruction on the day of discharge (Martens, 1998). In this regard, healthcare professionals have reported lack of time, delayed prescription writing by physicians, and being unaware of discharge plans as barriers to teaching (Martens, 1998; Alibhai, Han, &

Naglie, 1999). Short discharge notice may account for nurses' reports of spending only 2-15 minutes doing discharge medication teaching, often within 1-2 hours of discharge (Martens, 1998). In another study, physicians and pharmacists reported spending 13 or 14 minutes teaching patients about their medications, respectively (Alibhai et al., 1999). Hurried teaching by numerous professionals when patients and families are tired is likely to reduce older adults' abilities to integrate new information. This may contribute to the increased anxiety level reported by older adults on the day of discharge (Esposito, 1995). It makes sense to think that a hectic work environment (Vincent et al., 1998) could adversely affect professionals' abilities to plan and provide more comprehensive and individualized teaching given competing patient needs, sparse interdisciplinary communication and short discharge notice.

Additional factors contribute to limited medication teaching; healthcare professionals provided less discharge medication teaching to patients who were non-English speaking, were cognitively impaired, had no new medications, or had no perceived need (Alibhai et al., 1999). Here, one can draw a possible connection to outcomes: outpatients were more likely to experience drug complications if side effects had not been explained before treatment, their primary language was not English or Spanish, or they reported lower adherence (Gandhi et al., 2000). Paradoxically, those individuals not receiving medication instructions, such as non-English speaking patients, may be the ones who could benefit the most from individualized teaching. These situations reflect aspects of human error such as knowledge-based mistakes (Reason, 1990) when professionals overlook important factors (e.g., cognitive impairment) or do not apply relevant knowledge.

Issues and the Impact of Patient Non-Adherence

Accurately managing medications can be difficult for older adults. Non-adherence is a complex, multifaceted concept that is considered a possible medical error by some such as Barber (2002), who suggested using a human error framework (Reason, 1990) to examine the multiple factors contributing to patient non-adherence. Specifically, Barber (2002) advocated a shift in focus from individual patients to include their local environments and broader organizational issues as latent failures that inadvertently affect patient non-adherence. In some cases, patient non- adherence led to drug-related emergency room or hospital admissions (7.6%-12%) in Australia and India (Chan, Nicklason, & Vial, 2001; Malhotra, Karan, Pandhi, & Jain, 2001) and preventable

ADEs among older outpatients in the United States (Gurwitz et al., 2003). Patient non-adherence is discussed here because it may be avoidable when older adults' unique learning and fiscal needs are more properly assessed and plans are adjusted accordingly.

Among reasons for non-adherence, older adults reported missing doses because they forgot, changed to an unconventional treatment, or adjusted a dose to produce a desired response or to avoid side effects (Conn, Taylor, & Stineman, 1992; Malhotra et al., 2001). Although some older patients may sometimes avoid ADEs through non-adherence, chronically ill patients who take less medicine than prescribed may experience a decline in health (Heisler et al., 2004). Drug costs are another factor; older adults selectively fill prescriptions or intentionally skip doses (i.e., "stretching") because of the expense (Mitchell, Mathews, Hunt, Cobb, & Watson, 2001; Steinman, Sands, & Covinsky, 2001). The Medicare Discount Drug Cards are designed to address such concerns. Yet, in its early stage of implementation this program has generated confusion (Silberner, 2004) and further confounded an already complicated situation. The full implementation in 2006 promises to be far more confusing than the initial stage has been.

Education and cognitive function are related to medication adherence issues in elderly home care patients after hospital discharge (Gray et al., 2001). Older adults who were cognitively impaired and taking more medications tended to under-adhere (Gray et al., 2001). Not surprisingly, cognitively impaired older adults with complex regimens made more medication errors (Maddigan, Farris, Keating, Wiens, & Johnson, 2003). These findings are concerning when 54% of cognitively impaired older adults reported managing their own medications (Meyer & Schuna, 1989) and cognitive impairment can go undetected among elderly patients (Chodosh et al., 2004). These studies indicate that non-adherence likely includes elements of human error such as disruptions in medication routines or a failure to address a patient's limited comprehension (Vincent et al., 1998; Reason, 2002).

Medication-Related Risk Factors

The complexity of geriatric care places older adults at risk for medication-related problems. Studies have revealed that older adults who have multiple chronic conditions (i.e., > 6), take complex medication regimens (i.e., > 6 per day or > 12 doses/day), have cognitive impairment, or were recently transferred from a hospital were at greater risk for medication-related problems (Fouts, Hanlon, Pieper, Perfetto, &

Fienberg, 1997; Krska et al., 2001; Meredith et al., 2001; Gilbert, Roughead, Beilby, Mott, & Barratt, 2002; Sellors et al., 2003). Fouts and colleagues (1997) further characterized ADE risk in our frailest elders, adding as risk factors advanced age (i.e., > 85), prior adverse drug reaction history, physiologic measures (e.g., low body weight) and use of specific drugs (e.g., warfarin, digoxin). Other issues contributing to complex home medication regimens include irregular medication schedules, multiple prescribers and discontinued medication in patients' homes (Audette, Triller, Hamilton, & Briceland, 2002). These risk factors may be why some patients who take more medications tend to have a drug-related admission (Chan et al., 2001) or visit the emergency unit (Malhotra et al., 2001). From a human error perspective, overlooking these risk factors (e.g., co-morbidities) can contribute to ensuing medication problems (e.g., ADEs).

POTENTIAL SOLUTIONS

Although researchers have started to explore the dimensions of post-hospital home medication management problems, solutions are less well developed. Nolan (2000) advocated safer system designs that prevent errors, make errors visible or lessen their negative effects. Consistent with human error theory (Reason, 1990), Nolan outlined the need to reduce complexity, facilitate better information processing, employ technology, apply constraints and think of safety when making system changes. Applying this approach to post-hospital home medication management is especially challenging because of the logistics. Promising solutions that address fragmented care include active involvement of clinical pharmacists, interdisciplinary team development that extends continuous care beyond the hospital episode and informational strategies to improve hospital discharge processes, post-hospital care, patient outcomes and reduce costs.

Post-Hospital Transitional Care

Transitional care is a model that has demonstrated improved quality and cost outcomes among vulnerable older adults recently discharged from the hospital (Naylor et al., 1994; Naylor et al., 1999; Naylor et al., 2004; Smigelski et al., 2004). The transitional care intervention, provided by Advanced Practice Nurses (APNs), entails comprehensive and individualized care to older adults who are at risk for poor discharge outcomes (Naylor, 2000). A major focus of transitional care is the delivery of highly coordinated care and interdisciplinary collaboration that achieves quality and cost-effective care. This model emphasizes continuity of care (i.e., spanning hospital to home), comprehensive assessment and use of evidence-based guidelines to provide individualized, quality care that manages the complex and unique needs of older adults (Naylor, 2000). Specifically, three randomized clinical trials, funded by the National Institutes of Health, have consistently demonstrated improved quality and cost outcomes (Naylor et al., 1994; Naylor et al., 1999; Naylor et al., 2004). The most recent study detailed the APNs' interdisciplinary collaborative efforts to prevent functional decline, simplify medication regimens and focus on patient goals and teaching to promote adherence (Naylor et al., 2004). Study findings demonstrated an increased time to the first readmission, reduced total rehospitalizations and decreased total health care costs among elders with heart failure (Naylor et al., 2004). Additionally, preliminary findings from a secondary analysis, which is nearing completion, suggest that APNs' involvement improved adherence to evidence-based practice guidelines for older adults with heart failure and prevented potentially serious ADEs and medication errors during the vulnerable "handoff" from hospital to home (Schwartz, Naylor, Loh, & McCauley, 2004). These studies suggest that experienced and empowered interdisciplinary teams, placed correctly in the health care system, and working together to pro-actively manage complex older adults at home, can produce major cost savings and improve patient outcomes.

Roles of the Clinical Pharmacist

Numerous studies have shown the benefit of pharmacist involvement in the hospital and outpatient settings to improve prescribing, patient outcomes and decrease costs (Phillips & Carr-Lopez, 1990; Hanlon et al., 1996; Chiquette, Amato, & Bussey, 1998; Baran et al., 1999; Nathan, Goodyer, Lovejoy, & Rashid, 1999; Beney, Bero, & Bond, 2000; Krska et al., 2001; Gilbert et al., 2002; Sellors et al., 2003; Guignard, Couray-Targe, Colin, & Chamba, 2003; Isetts, Brown, Schondelmeyer, & Lenarz, 2003). Both patients and pharmacists have supported an expanded role of community pharmacists that includes counseling and disease management services (Baran et al., 1999; Volume, Farris, Kassam, Cox, & Cave, 2001). Community pharmacists performing medication reviews and providing interventions (e.g., counseling) improved patients' medication knowledge, and correct drug usage (Nathan et al., 1999; Krska et al., 2001), and may have prevented hospitalizations among older adults in the United Kingdom (Nathan et al., 1999). However, in other instances a lack of time, insufficient patient privacy, limited access to patient information (e.g., laboratory values), and inadequate communication between community pharmacists and physicians were reported barriers to providing more comprehensive services (Amsler et al., 2001). Making optimal use of the pharmacist requires actively including the pharmacist into the patient management team.

Pharmacists in the hospital can have greater opportunities to address medication problems. Hospital pharmacists who provided discharge medication teaching and contacted prescribers reduced the number of discharge medications and doses per day among complex patients (Calabrese et al., 2003) and such counseling has also improved patients' medication knowledge, adherence and was associated with fewer unplanned physician visits and hospital readmissions (Al-Rashed, Wright, Roebuck, Sunter, & Chrystyn, 2002). A hospital based "community services liaison pharmacist" in Northern Ireland demonstrated similar outcomes of reduced hospital readmission rates and improved home medication management among older adults taking four or more medications (Brookes, Scott, & McConnell, 2000). In an ensuing study, community liaison pharmacists significantly reduced medication discrepancies, improved patient knowledge and they identified medication-related problems that were often due to omissions (Bolas, Brookes, Scott, & McElnay, 2004).

Pharmacists on Interdisciplinary Teams

Pharmacist participation on multidisciplinary teams has led to fewer preventable ADEs in hospitals (Leape et al., 1999) and better post-hospital outcomes (Hawe & Higgins, 1990; Alibhai et al., 1999; Brookes et al., 2000; Dudas, Bookwalter, Kerr, & Pantilat, 2001; Al-Rashed et al., 2002; Calabrese et al., 2003; Triller, Clause, Briceland, & Hamilton, 2003). In the same way, better communication between prescribers and clinical pharmacists (Gurwitz et al., 2003) may prevent ADEs in the community due to poor communication (Gandhi et al., 2003). Boling (2002) has advocated use of a home care pharmacist consultant because of the heterogeneity of home care situations and the significant issues of discontinuity between settings and providers.

Home care consultation and in-home pharmacist visits have improved medication use, reducing discrepancies, therapeutic duplications and unnecessary medications among elderly home care patients (Hsia Der et al., 1997; Meredith et al., 2002; Triller et al., 2003). Pharmacists' interventions included providing educational materials about managing specific medication problems to the home care nurses, assessing drug utilization through patient chart reviews, in-home visits and/or telephone conversations, and consulting in care conferences (Brown et al., 1998; Meredith et al., 2002; Triller et al., 2003). Meredith et al. (2002) targeted specific high-risk medication problems such as unnecessary duplication and cardiovascular medication problems with an evidence-based model that has subsequently been tested in four home care agencies and demonstrated multiple benefits to patients, nurses and home care administrators and managers (Frey & Rahman, 2003).

Older adults in other settings may also benefit from similar interventions. A medication review by an interdisciplinary team (i.e., physician, nurse and clinical pharmacist) resulted in fewer medications and cost-savings to a group of community-dwelling older adults; however, this resource-intensive intervention was not considered cost-effective (Williams et al., 2004). In contrast, consultant pharmacists reviewing drug regimens of high-risk older adults in U.S. nursing homes are estimated to save approximately $3.6 billion annually in costs secondary to medication-related problems and improve therapeutic outcomes (Bootman, Harrison, & Cox, 1997). These studies underscore the importance of creating cost-effective interventions to improve patient outcomes among high-risk older adults.

Informational Technologies

Informational technologies may also help to improve post-hospital home medication management. Discharge prescriptions tended to be more accurate and had fewer duplications and omissions when pharmacists generated computerized discharge orders, which were subsequently reviewed and authorized by the physician (Chantelois & Suzuki, 2003). Hospital discharge prescription forms improved communication with local pharmacies that led to fewer omissions, proper discontinuation by community pharmacist of medications stopped in the hospital and increased consistency of medication profiles (Paquette-Lamontagne, McLean, Besse, & Cusson, 2001).

Future Research

In addition to these efforts, research is needed to explore transition-specific medication problems among vulnerable older adults, and to test possible solutions. Hospitalized older adults could benefit from better planning and teaching about their post-hospital home medication regimens that are individualized to their needs, abilities and resources. As such, research is needed to test hospital discharge and home follow-up strategies targeted to lessen ADEs, therapeutic duplications, unplanned hospital admissions, emergency room visits and improve patient adherence. Interdisciplinary teamwork is essential in post-hospital medication management because the patient's care inevitably involves nurses, physicians and pharmacists; failure to function as a team in such complex scenarios is inherently dangerous.

CONCLUSION

Human error theory (Reason, 1990) helps us to identify factors contributing to problems of post-hospital home medication management among older adults. Hospital discharge medication practices are poorly designed, inefficient and prone to errors. Hospitals are hectic, distracting environments for professionals and older adults alike that allow little time to plan optimal medication management and address individual learning needs. The fragmented system is vulnerable to medication errors such as undetected omissions, therapeutic duplications and discrepancies that are compounded by few inter-institutional feedback mechanisms and fragile communication.

The policy implications of involving pharmacists more integrally in post-hospital home health care are complex. Nursing homes, which serve a similar patient population, have extensive, mandatory involvement of pharmacists. If this service is valuable in nursing homes, why would it be any less so in home care? However, adopting such a strategy would require a significant change in home health care policy that would have to be matched with an appropriate change in funding. We are spending hundreds of billions of dollars each year developing, testing, marketing, and purchasing drugs. We also expended an estimated 177 billion in 2000 for care associated with drug-related morbidity and mortality (Ernst & Grizzle, 2001). It is only reasonable that a proportionate investment be made in safe medication practices for vulnerable, high-risk older adults.

REFERENCES

Adams, K., & Corrigan, J. M. (2003). *Priority areas for national action: Transforming health care quality.* Washington, DC: National Academies Press.

Al-Rashed, S. A., Wright, D. J., Roebuck, N., Sunter, W., & Chrystyn, H. (2002). The value of inpatient pharmaceutical counselling to elderly patients prior to discharge. *British Journal of Clinical Pharmacology, 54*(6), 657-64.

Alibhai, S. M., Han, R. K., & Naglie, G. (1999). Medication education of acutely hospitalized older patients. *Journal of General Internal Medicine, 14*(10), 610-6.

Amsler, M. R., Murray, M. D., Tierney, W. M., Brewer, N., Harris, L. E., Marrero, D. G. & Weinberger, M. (2001). Pharmaceutical care in chain pharmacies: Beliefs and attitudes of pharmacists and patients. *Journal of the American Pharmacology Association (Wash), 41*(6), 850-5.

Audette, C. M., Triller, D. M., Hamilton, R., & Briceland, L. L. (2002). Classifying drug-related problems in home care. *American Journal of Health-Systems Pharmacy, 59,* 2407-9.

Baran, R. W., Crumlish, K., Patterson, H., Shaw, J., Erwin, W. G., Wylie, J. D., & Duong, P. (1999). Improving outcomes of community-dwelling older patients with diabetes through pharmacist counseling. *American Journal of Health-System Pharmacy, 56,* 1535-9.

Barber, N. (2002). Should we consider non-compliance a medical error? *Quality & Safety in Health Care, 11*(1), 81-4.

Bates, D. W., Boyle, D. L., Vander Vliet, M. B., Schneider, J., & Leape, L. (1995). Relationship between medication errors and adverse drug events. *Journal of General Internal Medicine, 10*(4), 199-205.

Bates, D. W., Cullen, D. J., Laird, N., Petersen, L. A., Small, S. D., Servi, D., Laffel, G., Sweitzer, B. J., Shea, B. F., Hallisey, R. et al. (1995). Incidence of adverse drug events and potential adverse drug events. Implications for prevention. ADE Prevention Study Group. *Journal of the American Medical Association, 274*(1), 29-34.

Bedell, S. E., Jabbour, S., Goldberg, R., Glaser, H., Gobble, S., Young-Xu, Y., Graboys, T. B., & Ravid, S. (2000). Discrepancies in the use of medications: Their extent and predictors in an outpatient practice. *Archives of Internal Medicine, 160*(14), 2129-34.

Beers, M. H., Sliwkowski, J., & Brooks, J. (1992). Compliance with medication orders among the elderly after hospital discharge. *Hospital Formulary, 27*(7), 720-4.

Beney, J., Bero, L. A., & Bond, C. (2000). Expanding the roles of outpatient pharmacists: Effects on health services utilisation, costs, and patient outcomes. *Cochrane Database Systematic Review,* (3), CD000336.

Bogner, M.S. (1994). Introduction. In M.S. Bogner (Ed.), *Human error in medicine* (pp.1-11). Hillsdale, NJ: Lawrence Erlbaum Associates Inc.

Bolas, H., Brookes, K., Scott, M., & McElnay, J. (2004). Evaluation of a hospital-based community liaison pharmacy service in Northern Ireland. *Pharmacy World Science, 26*(2), 114-20.

Boling, P. A. (2002). Strategic use of home care pharmacy consultation may be worthwhile. *Journal of the American Geriatrics Society, 50*(9), 1597-8.

Boockvar, K., Fishman, E., Kyriacou, C. K., Monias, A., Gavi, S., & Cortes, T. (2004). Adverse events due to discontinuations in drug use and dose changes in patients transferred between acute and long-term care facilities. *Archives of Internal Medicine, 164*(5), 545-50.

Bootman, J. L., Harrison, D. L., & Cox, E. (1997). The health care cost of drug-related morbidity and mortality in nursing facilities. *Archives of Internal Medicine, 157*(18), 2089-96.

Brennan, T. A., Leape, L. L., Laird, N. M., Hebert, L., Localio, A. R., Lawthers, A. G., Newhouse, J. P., Weiler, P. C., & Hiatt, H. H. (1991). Incidence of adverse events and negligence in hospitalized patients. Results of the Harvard Medical Practice Study I. *New England Journal of Medicine, 324*(6), 370-6.

Brookes, K., Scott, M. G., & McConnell, J. B. (2000). The benefits of a hospital based community services liaison pharmacist. *Pharmacy World Science, 22*(2), 33-8.

Brown, N. J., Griffin, M.R., Ray, W. A., Meredith, S., Beers, M. H., Marren, J., Robles, M., Stergachis, A., Wood, J. J., & Avorn, J. (1998). A model for improving medication use in home health care. *Journal of the American Pharmaceutical Association, 38*, 696-702.

Calabrese, A. T., Cholka, K., Lenhart, S. E., McCarty, B., Zewe, G., Sunseri, D., Roberts, M., & Kapoor, W. (2003). Pharmacist involvement in a multidisciplinary inpatient medication education program. *American Journal of Health-System Pharmacy, 60*(10), 1012-8.

Chan, C. Y., Maxwell, P. R., Koger, C. A., Gamboa, C. D., & Brewer, J. G. (1990). Screening discharge prescriptions on a pediatric ward. *American Journal of Hospital Pharmacy, 47*(9), 2060-1.

Chan, M., Nicklason, F., & Vial, J. H. (2001). Adverse drug events as a cause of hospital admission in the elderly. *Internal Medicine Journal, 31*(4), 199-205.

Chantelois, E. P., & Suzuki, N. T. (2003). A pilot program comparing physician- and pharmacist-ordered discharge medications at a Veterans Affairs medical center. *American Journal of Health-System Pharmacy, 60*(16), 1652-6.

Chiquette, E., Amato, M. G., & Bussey, H. I. (1998). Comparison of an anticoagulation clinic with usual medical care: Anticoagulation control, patient outcomes, and health care costs. *Archives of Internal Medicine, 158*(15), 1641-7.

Chodosh, J., Petitti, D. B., Elliott, M., Hays, R. D., Crooks, V. C., Reuben, D. B., Galen Buckwalter, J., & Wenger, N. (2004). Physician recognition of cognitive impairment: Evaluating the need for improvement. *Journal of the American Geriatrics Society, 52*(7), 1051-9.

Coleman, E. A. (2003). Falling through the cracks: Challenges and opportunities for improving transitional care for persons with continuous complex care needs. *Journal of the American Geriatrics Society, 51*(4), 549-55.

Conn, V., Taylor, S. G., & Stineman, A. (1992). Medication management by recently hospitalized older adults. *Journal of Community Health Nursing, 9*(1), 1-11.

Cook, R. I., Render, M., & Woods, D. D. (2000). Gaps in the continuity of care and progress on patient safety. *British Medical Journal, 320,*, 791-4.

Creditor, M. C. (1993). Hazards of hospitalization of the elderly. *Annals of Internal Medicine, 118*(3), 219-23.

Doucet, J., Jego, A., Geffory, C. E., Capet, C., Couffin, E., Fauchais, A. L., Chassagne, P., Mouton-Schleifer, D., & Bercoft, E. (2002). Preventable and non-preventable risk factors for adverse drug events related to hospital admission in the elderly. *Clinical Drug Investigations, 22*(6), 385-392.

Dudas, V., Bookwalter, T., Kerr, K. M., & Pantilat, S. Z. (2001). The impact of follow-up telephone calls to patients after hospitalization. *American Journal of Medicine, 111*(9B), 26S-30S.

Ernst, F. R., & Grizzle, A. J. (2001). Drug-related morbidity and mortality: Updating the Cost-of-illness model. *Journal of the American Pharmaceutical Association, 41*(2), 192-199.

Esposito, L. (1995). The effects of medication education on adherence to medication regimens in an elderly population. *Journal of Advanced Nursing, 21*(5), 935-43.

Forster, A. J., Clark, H. D., Menard, A., Dupuis, N., Chernish, R., Chandok, N., Khan, A., & van Walraven, C. (2004). Adverse events among medical patients after discharge from hospital. *Canadian Medical Association Journal, 170*(3), 345-9.

Forster, A. J., Murff, H. J., Peterson, J. F., Gandhi, T. K., & Bates, D. W. (2003). The incidence and severity of adverse events affecting patients after discharge from the hospital. *Annals of Internal Medicine, 138*(3), 161-7.

Fouts, M., Hanlon, J., Pieper, C., Perfetto, E., & Fienberg, J. (1997). Identification of elderly nursing facility residents at high risk for drug-related problems. *Consultant Pharmacist, 12*, 1103-1111.

Frey, D. & Rahman, A. (2003). Medication management: An evidence-based model that decreases adverse events. *Home Healthcare Nurse, 21*(6), 404-412.

Gandhi, T. K., Burstin, H. R., Cook, E. F., Puopolo, A. L., Haas, J. S., Brennan, T. A., & Bates, D. W. (2000). Drug complications in outpatients. *Journal of General Internal Medicine, 15*(3), 149-54.

Gandhi, T. K., Weingart, S. N., Borus, J., Seger, A. C., Peterson, J., Burdick, E., Seger, D. L., Shu, K., Federico, F., Leape, L. L., & Bates, D. W. (2003). Adverse drug events in ambulatory care. *New England Journal of Medicine, 348*(16), 1556-64.

Gilbert, A. L., Roughead, E. E., Beilby, J., Mott, K., & Barratt, J. D. (2002). Collaborative medication management services: Improving patient care. *The Medical Journal of Australia, 177*(4), 189-92.

Gray, S. L., Mahoney, J. E., & Blough, D. K. (1999). Adverse drug events in elderly patients receiving home health services following hospital discharge. *Annals of Pharmacotherapy, 33*(11), 1147-53.

Gray, S. L., Mahoney, J. E., & Blough, D. K. (2001). Medication adherence in elderly patients receiving home health services following hospital discharge. *Annals of Pharmacotherapy, 35*(5), 539-45.

Guignard, A. P., Couray-Targe, S., Colin, C., & Chamba, G. (2003). Economic impact of pharmacists' interventions with nonsteroidal antiinflammatory drugs. *Annals of Pharmacotherapy, 37*(3), 332-8.

Gurwitz, J. H., & Avorn, J. (1991). The ambiguous relationship between aging and Adverse drug reactions. *Annals of Internal Medicine, 114*(11), 956-966.

Gurwitz, J. H., Field, T. S., Harrold, L. R., Rothschild, J., Debellis, K., Seger, A. C., Cadoret, C., Fish, L. S., Garber, L., Kelleher, M., & Bates, D. W. (2003). Incidence and preventability of adverse drug events among older persons in the ambulatory setting. *Journal of the American Medical Association, 289*(9), 1107-16.

Gurwitz, J. H. & Rochon, P. (2002). Improving the quality of medication use in elderly patients: A not-so-simple prescription. *Archives of Internal Medicine, 162*(15), 1670-2

Hanlon, J. T., Artz, M. B., Pieper, C. F., Lindblad, C. I., Sloane, R. J., Ruby, C. M., & Schmader, K.E. (2004). Inappropriate medication use among frail elderly inpatients. *Annals of Pharmacotherapy, 38*(1), 9-14.

Hanlon, J. T., Weinberger, M., Samsa, G. P., Schmader, K. E., Uttech, K. M., Lewis, I. K., Cowper, P. A., Landsman, P. B., Cohen, H. J., & Feussner, J. R. (1996). A randomized, controlled trial of a clinical pharmacist intervention to improve inappropriate prescribing in elderly outpatients with polypharmacy. *American Journal of Medicine, 100*(4), 428-37.

Hawe, P., & Higgins, G. (1990). Can medication education improve the drug compliance of the elderly? Evaluation of an in hospital program. *Patient Education and Counseling, 16*(2), 151-60.

Heisler, M., Langa, K. M., Eby, E. L., Fendrick, A. M., Kabeto, M. U., & Piette, J. D. (2004). The health effects of restricting prescription medication use because of cost. *Medical Care, 42*(7), 626-634.

Hsia Der, E., Rubenstein, L. Z., & Choy, G. S. (1997). The benefits of in-home pharmacy evaluation for older persons. *Journal of the American Geriatrics Society, 45*(2), 211-4.

Isetts, B. J., Brown, L. M., Schondelmeyer, S. W., & Lenarz, L. A. (2003). Quality assessment of a collaborative approach for decreasing drug-related morbidity and achieving therapeutic goals. *Archives of Internal Medicine, 163*(15), 1813-20.

Juurlink, D. N., Mamdani, M., Kopp, A., Laupacis, A., & Redelmeier, D. A. (2003). Drug-drug interactions among elderly patients hospitalized for drug toxicity. *Journal of the American Medical Association, 289*(13), 1652-8.

Kohn, L. T., Corrigan, J. M., & Donaldson, M. S. (2000). *To Err is Human: Building a safer health system.* Washington, DC: National Academy Press.

Krska, J., Cromarty, J. A., Arris, F., Jamieson, D., Hansford, D., Duffus, P. R., Downie, G., & Seymour, D. G. (2001). Pharmacist-led medication review in patients over 65: A randomized, controlled trial in primary care. *Age and Ageing, 30*(3), 205-11.

Leape, L.L. (1994). The preventability of medical errors. In M.S. Bogner (Ed.), Human error in medicine (pp. 13-25). Hillsdale, NJ: Lawrence Erlbaum Associates, Inc.

Leape, L. L., Bates, D. W., Cullen, D. J., Cooper, J., Demonaco, H. J., Gallivan, T., Hallisey, R., Ives, J., Laird, N., Laffel, G. et al. (1995). Systems analysis of adverse drug events. ADE Prevention Study Group. *Journal of the American Medical Association, 274*(1), 35-43.

Leape, L. L., Brennan, T. A., Laird, N., Lawthers, A. G., Localio, A. R., Barnes, B. A., Hebert, L., Newhouse, J. P., Weiler, P. C., & Hiatt, H. (1991). The nature of adverse events in hospitalized patients. Results of the Harvard Medical Practice Study II. *New England Journal of Medicine, 324*(6), 377-84.

Leape, L. L., Cullen, D. J., Clapp, M. D., Burdick, E., Demonaco, H. J., Erickson, J. I., & Bates, D. W. (1999). Pharmacist participation on physician rounds and adverse drug events in the intensive care unit. *Journal of the American Medical Association, 282*(3), 267-70.

Lewis, D., Pavlis, B., Chen, J., & Fields, S. D. (2004). Medication discrepancies during the transition to home health care in the elderly. [Abstract] *Journal of the American Geriatrics Society, 52(4S)*, S193.

Maddigan, S. L., Farris, K. B., Keating, N., Wiens, C. A., & Johnson, J. A. (2003). Predictors of older adults' capacity for medication management in a self-medication program: A retrospective chart review. *Journal of Aging and Health, 15*(2), 332-52.

Malhotra, S., Karan, R. S., Pandhi, P., & Jain, S. (2001). Drug-related medical emergencies in the elderly: Role of adverse drug reactions and non-compliance. *Postgraduate Medicine Journal, 77*(913), 703-7.

Martens, K. H. (1998). An ethnographic study of the process of medication discharge education (MDE). *Journal of Advanced Nursing, 27*(2), 341-8.

McDonnell, P. J., & Jacobs, M. R. (2002). Hospital admissions resulting from preventable adverse drug reactions. *Annals of Pharmacotherapy, 36*(9), 1331-6.

Meredith, S., Feldman, P., Frey, D., Giammarco, L., Hall, K., Arnold, K., Brown, N. J., & Ray, W. A. (2002). Improving medication use in newly admitted home healthcare patients: A randomized controlled trial. *Journal of the American Geriatrics Society, 50*(9), 1484-91.

Meyer, M. E., & Schuna, A. A. (1989). Assessment of geriatric patients' functional ability to take medication. *DICP: The annals of pharmacotherapy, 23*(2), 171-4.

Mitchell, J., Mathews, H. F., Hunt, L. M., Cobb, K. H., & Watson, R. W. (2001). Mismanaging prescription medications among rural elders: The effects of socioeconomic status, health status, and medication profile indicators. *Gerontologist, 41*(3), 348-56.

Moore, C., Wisnivesky, J., Williams, S., & McGinn, T. (2003). Medical errors related to discontinuity of care from an inpatient to an outpatient setting. *Journal of General Internal Medicine, 18*(8), 646-51.

Morrill, G. B., & Barreuther, C. (1988). Screening discharge prescriptions. *American Journal Hospital Pharmacy, 45*(9), 1904-5.

Nathan, A., Goodyer, L., Lovejoy, A., & Rashid, A. (1999). 'Brown bag' medication reviews as a means of optimizing patients' use of medication and of identifying potential clinical problems. *Family Practice, 16*(3), 278-82.

Naylor, M. D. (2000). A decade of transitional care research with vulnerable elders. *Journal of Cardiovascular Nursing, 14*(3), 1-14.

Naylor, M. D., Brooten, D. A., Campbell, R. L., Maislin, G., McCauley, K. M., & Schwartz, J. S. (2004). Transitional care of older adults hospitalized with heart failure: A randomized, controlled trial. *Journal of the American Geriatrics Society, 52*(5), 675-84.

Naylor, M. D., Brooten, D., Campbell, R., Jacobsen, B. S., Mezey, M. D., Pauly, M. V., & Schwartz, J. S. (1999). Comprehensive discharge planning and home follow-up of hospitalized elders: A randomized clinical trial. *Journal of the American Medical Association, 281*(7), 613-620.

Naylor, M. D., Brooten, D., Jones, R., Lavizzo-Mourey, R., Mezey, M., & Pauly, M. (1994). Comprehensive discharge planning for the hospitalized elderly: A randomized clinical trial. *Annals of Internal Medicine, 120*, 999-1006.

Nolan, T. W. (2000). System changes to improve patient safety. *British Medical Journal, 320,* 771-3.

Paquette-Lamontagne, N., McLean, W. M., Besse, L., & Cusson, J. (2001). Evaluation of a new integrated discharge prescription form. *Annals of Pharmacotherapy, 35*(7-8), 953-8.

Phillips, S. L., & Carr-Lopez, S. M. (1990). Impact of a pharmacist on medication discontinuation in a hospital-based geriatric clinic. *American Journal of Hospital Pharmacy, 47*(5), 1075-9.

Reason, J. (1990). *Human Error.* Cambridge, UK: Cambridge University Press.

Reason, J. (1995). Understanding adverse events: Human factors. *Quality Health Care, 4*(2), 80-9.

Reason, J. (2002). Combating omission errors through task analysis and good reminders. *Quality & Safety in Health Care, 11*(1), 40-4.

Rothschild, J. M., Bates, D. W., & Leape, L. L. (2000). Preventable medical injuries in older patients. *Archives of Internal Medicine, 160*(18), 2717-28.

Rozich, J. D., & Resar, R. K. (2001). Medication safety: One organization's approach to the challenge. *Journal of Clinical Outcomes Management, 8*(10), 27-34.

Schumock, G. T., Guenette, A. J., Keys, T. V., & Hutchinson, R. A. (1994). Prescribing errors for patients about to be discharged from a university teaching hospital. *American Journal of Hospital Pharmacy, 51*(18), 2288, 2290.

Schwartz, S. J., Naylor, M. D., Loh, E., & McCauley, K. (2004). [Physician-Nurse Co-Management of Elders with Heart Failure]. Unpublished raw data.

Sellors, J., Kaczorowski, J., Sellors, C., Dolovich, L., Woodward, C., Willan, A., Goeree, R., Cosby, R., Trim, K., Sebaldt, R., Howard, M., Hardcastle, L., & Poston, J. (2003). A randomized controlled trial of a pharmacist consultation program for family physicians and their elderly patients. *Canadian Medical Association Journal, 169*(1), 17-22.

Silberner, J. (2004) *Puzzling Through Medicare's Discount Cards* [Web Page]. URL http://www.npr.org/features/feature.php?wfId=1901388 [2004, May 23].

Smigelski, C. W., Hungate, B., & Boling, P. A. (2004). Transitional model of care: Bridging inpatient and outpatient care. [Abstract] *Journal of the American Geriatrics Society, 52*(4), S194-5.

Steinman, M. A., Sands, L. P., & Covinsky, K. E. (2001). Self-restriction of medications due to cost in seniors without prescription coverage. *Journal of General Internal Medicine, 16*(12), 793-9.

Triller, D. M., Clause, S. L., Briceland, L. L., & Hamilton, R. A. (2003). Resolution of drug-related problems in home care patients through a pharmacy referral service. *American Journal of Health-System Pharmacy, 60,* 905-910.

Tsilimingras, D., Rosen, A. K., & Berlowitz, D. R. (2003). Review article: Patient safety in geriatrics: A call for action. *Journal of Gerontology A Biological Science, Medical Science, 58*(9), M813-9.

Vincent, C., Taylor-Adams, S., Chapman, E. J., Hewett, D., Prior, S., Strange, P., & Tizzard, A. (2000). How to investigate and analyse clinical incidents: Clinical risk unit and association of litigation and risk management protocol. *British Medical Journal, 320,* 777-781.

Vincent, C., Taylor-Adams, S., & Stanhope, N. (1998). Framework for analysing risk and safety in clinical medicine. *British Medical Journal, 316*, 1154-7.

Volume, C. I., Farris, K. B., Kassam, R., Cox, C. E., & Cave, A. (2001). Pharmaceutical care research and education project: Patient outcomes. *Journal of the American Pharmacology Association (Wash), 41* (3), 411-20.

Williams, M. E., Pulliam, C. C., Hunter, R., Johnson, T. M., Owens, J. E., Kincaid, J., Porter, C., & Koch, G. (2004). The short-term effect of interdisciplinary medication review on function and cost in ambulatory elderly people. *Journal of the American Geriatrics Society, 52*(1), 93-8.

Risk of Medication Errors
at Hospital Discharge
and Barriers to Problem Resolution

Susan M. Enguidanos, MPH, PhD
Richard D. Brumley, MD

SUMMARY. Medication errors are common among older adults, particularly among those who are at heightened risk due to transfer between care settings. Determining accurate medications for hospitalized patients is a complicated process. This paper presents findings from a small pilot study conducted to identify medication documentation problems at the point of hospital discharge among older adults and the problems encountered in developing new technological systems to address these problems. A prospective study was conducted within a managed care medical center that included patient and physician surveys and chart reviews. A review of 104 medical records revealed several problems in the documentation of patient medication including legibility, use of medical abbreviations and incomplete and missing entries. While patients overall were satisfied with medications communication efforts at discharge, physicians surveyed reported that these methods were inadequate in transmitting medication lists to primary care physicians, patients and other care providers. Patients reported taking more drugs than what were

Susan M. Enguidanos is Research Director at the Partners in Care Foundation. Richard D. Brumley is Medical Director at Home Health and Palliative Care, Southern California Permanente Medical Group, Kaiser Permanente TriCentral Service Area.

[Haworth co-indexing entry note]: "Risk of Medication Errors at Hospital Discharge and Barriers to Problem Resolution." Enguidanos, Susan M., and Richard D. Brumley. Co-published simultaneously in *Home Health Care Services Quarterly* (The Haworth Press, Inc.) Vol. 24, No. 1/2, 2005, pp. 123-135; and: *Improving Medication Management in Home Care: Issues and Solutions* (ed: Dennnee Frey) The Haworth Press, Inc., 2005, pp. 123-135. Single or multiple copies of this article are available for a fee from The Haworth Document Delivery Service [1-800-HAWORTH, 9:00 a.m. - 5:00 p.m. (EST). E-mail address: docdelivery@haworthpress.com].

listed in the medical record. These findings led to the development, testing, and implementation of an electronic medication sheet. Despite the success in developing this new system, few physicians engaged in its use, with most preferring to continue with their standard discharge practices of written communication. *[Article copies available for a fee from The Haworth Document Delivery Service: 1-800-HAWORTH. E-mail address: <docdelivery@haworthpress.com> Website: <http://www.HaworthPress.com>*
© *2005 by The Haworth Press, Inc. All rights reserved.]*

KEYWORDS. Medication errors, hospital discharge, care transition, older adults, electronic medication record

INTRODUCTION

Although seniors represent a small segment of the U.S. population, they consume one-third of all prescription drugs and purchase nearly half of all the over-the-counter medications sold (Kahl, 1992). Medication related problems have been estimated to be a leading cause of death for hospitalized patients (Kohn, Corrigan, & Donaldson, 1999). Errors in medications are ranked as the fifth leading cause of death for people over the age of 65 (Lazarou, Pomeranz, & Corey, 1998). In 1994, an estimated 106,000 hospital patients died in the U.S. as a result of adverse drug events (Lazarou et al., 1998). The elderly, in particular, are the most susceptible to medications errors. They are more likely to experience a side effect to the medication, have decreased organ functioning which results in delayed metabolism of drugs, have an increased number of chronic conditions requiring multiple medications, and have potentially multiple prescribing physicians. All of these contribute to their increased sensitivity to medications (Mark H. Beers, 2000-2001; Larsen & Hoot Martin, 1999).

Among a general population of adults, Bates et al. (1995) found that 6.5 of every 100 hospital admissions were due to adverse drug events and an additional 5.5 of every 100 had the potential for an adverse drug event. Many of these prescription medication errors are avoidable; 7.3 adverse drug events per 100 admissions were preventable (out of a total of 12 current and potential per 100 admissions).

Transfer between levels of care offers opportunities for increased risk of medication errors (Beers, Sliwkowski, & Brooks, 1992). In a pilot study examining the transfer of information between the hospital and a rehabilitation unit, 13% of the discharge summaries failed to include a list of the patient's current medications. Of those that did list medications, 59% were inaccurate (Sobel, Medina-Walpole, & Katz, 2004). These data illustrate an alarming possibility for medication error. Additionally, emergency room visits and hospital admissions oftentimes result in medication additions and changes. About 40% of older adults discharged from the emergency room have new prescriptions (Hedges et al., 1992). Moreover, among older adults discharged from the emergency room with at least one new prescription, the complexity of their daily medication regimen more than doubled for nearly half of the sample following addition of the new drug (Hayes, 1999). The study also reported that patient's knowledge of their medication instructions decreased as the complexity of their prescribed medications increased. Thus the transfer between care settings are associated with increased odds of medication errors. Lesar and colleagues (1997) found that the number of hospital admissions accounted for 83% of the variance in errors per 1000 patient-days (Lesar, Briceland, & Stein, 1997).

Medication errors are further exacerbated by incomplete, inaccurate, and illegible medication orders communicated to patients at the time of hospital discharge. Hospitalizations frequently involve new or altered medication prescriptions for patients. These changes in prescription medications are not always clearly communicated with patients and their caregivers at the time of discharge (Paparella, 2004). Further, medication errors are also increased by the use of medical terminology on patient documents. Medical lingo, such as "bid" (twice per day), "hs" (at bedtime), and "prn" (as needed) are frequently unknown by most individuals, furthering confusing issues around medication regimens. As a result, patients often experience frustration and confusion regarding their medication regimen. Of greater concern are the situations where patients inadvertently continue medications that have been discontinued or fail to continue or begin medication regimens due to inadequate communication practices at the time of hospital discharge. Finally, it is not uncommon for discharge orders to simply state, "continue current medications," sometimes after listing a new dose of an existing medication, which may lead the patient to believe that two different doses of the same medication must be taken.

The incidence of medication errors is not only due to misunderstandings between patient and providers but among sites of care as well. These same problems are experienced daily for patients who are discharged from the hospital to other service programs, such as skilled nursing facilities, home health agencies, long term care facilities and hospice programs. In a study of records of patients transferring from the acute care setting to a subacute unit, Johnson and colleagues (Johnson, Christmas, & Dunne, 2004) found that 70% of all transfer orders had at least one medication error, and nearly two thirds had 2 or more errors. Moreover, among medication errors at transfer from the hospital to nursing home, 20% resulted in adverse drug events (Boockvar et al., 2004). Medication regimens also are not communicated to the patients' primary care physician at the time of hospital discharge.

With the large numbers of patients discharged from the hospital each day, the risks of medication errors resulting from inadequate communication and documentation of needed medications are staggering (Coleman, 2003). Hospitalists (inpatient physicians) who may have only seen the patient for a day or two have the responsibility of determining proper medications including those not related to the recent hospitalization. These physicians face a multitude of challenges given the lack of centralization of medication prescribing and filling patterns.

The purpose of this paper is to present findings from an investigation of communication patterns regarding patient medications at discharge. Specifically, this paper will present findings from physician and patient survey as well as a review of medication orders of a random sample of older adults at hospital discharge. Additionally, this article will report on efforts made to improve medication communication at hospital discharge and outcomes associated with these efforts.

METHODS

This is a prospective study to determine the adequacy of medication communication patterns for older adults at the point of hospital discharge. The project was reviewed and approved by the medical facility's Institutional Review Board (IRB). As designated by the IRB, all potential participants were sent a letter advising them of the study and their rights to refuse to be interviewed.

A random sample of 104 patients over the age of 65 discharged from a large managed care medical center in Southern California was selected for review. The medication list from each of these patient charts was obtained and reviewed to determine the legibility, completeness, and the frequency of medical terminology use in communicating medication instructions to older patients. These medication lists are the sole source of information provided to patients by the hospital regarding their medication regimens to be followed at discharge. In addition, these patients were surveyed by telephone within three days of discharge to determine their satisfaction with the discharge medication instructions they received. Furthermore, 50 primary care and outpatient physicians with medical center admitting privileges were surveyed regarding their satisfaction with discharge instructions and the medication record.

Instruments

Chart Review. The discharge medication orders were extracted from each patient chart and reviewed to determine (1) completeness, (2) legibility, and (3) use of medical terminology. A data collection form was developed to track the number of medications listed and the extent of the problems in each patient document.

Physician Survey. An 8-item physician survey was developed to measure the level of communication between the primary care physician and the medical center following the discharge of primary care physicians' patients regarding medication orders. The survey sought to measure the frequency of communication between the hospital and the primary care physician regarding patient medications following hospital discharge, primary care physician satisfaction with the quality of these communications, and physician perception of the quality of the communication between the hospital and their patient. This survey was developed as an online questionnaire and e-mailed to physicians with admitting privileges in the medial center and/or the primary care physicians for patients admitted to the medical center.

Patient Survey. A 13-item survey was developed to measure patient satisfaction with the discharge instructions they received at the time they left the hospital. This survey measured the extent of patient perceived clarity on the communication regarding medications at the point of hospital discharge. Trained research assistants conducted this interview via telephone within three days of hospital discharge.

Analyses

All data was entered and stored in SPSS 10.1 statistical software package. Descriptive analyses were conducted on all variables. For comparisons of differences between patient reported number of medications and number of medications listed in the medical record on the discharge sheet, a paired sample t-test was conducted. Alpha was set at .05.

RESULTS

A total of 104 older patients were surveyed and medication sheets reviewed. About half (51%) were male and age ranged from 66 to 97 years (M = 76.3, SD = 7.3). Most interviews (73%) were conducted directly with the patient, 15% of interviews were with the spouse, 9% with the child, and 3% with other relative/caregiver. Overall, patients reported taking from 0 to 19 medications, with an average of 5.6 (SD = 4.1) medications taken.

Patient Satisfaction

Overall, patients reported high rates of agreement in terms of medication communication practices at the time of discharge. About 82% of the respondents were clear about the medications they should be taking and 89% agreed that discharge instructions were clearly explained (see Table 1). However, patients were less enthusiastic in their support of the overall level of information they received at hospital discharge, with only 40% strongly agreeing that information received was easy to understand. Further, only 59% strongly agreed that the medication sheet they received at discharge was complete.

Chart Reviews

Of the 104 patients identified for chart reviews, charts were located for 80. Of the 80 medical charts reviewed, medication sheets were found for 73 (91%). About 18% (14) of the medication sheets simply indicated "continue current medications" (see Figure 1). Of the remaining 66 records listing medications, 29% had illegible entries in the medication list (see Figure 2), and 56% had missing entries, primarily in the section indicating reason for taking the medication. Further, 23% of the entries contained medical terminology such as "prn," "sq," "po" and "q" (see Figure 3).

Most notable was the discrepancy in convergence between the number of medications reported by the patient versus the number listed in the chart. Only six cases matched in terms of number of medications reported by patients and medications listed on the medication sheet. The average number of medications listed in the hospital record was 4.31 (SD = 2.96) as compared to 6.33 (SD = 4.24) reported by the patient (t = 3.4, p = .001).

TABLE 1. Patient Satisfaction with Discharge Communication

Question	Strongly Agree (%)
I know when to take my medications:	94%
Discharge instructions were communicated to me using language I understand:	89%
I know what each of my medications is for:	88%
I am clear about which medications I should be taking:	82%
I had no difficulty reading or understanding the instruction and medication sheet I received at discharge:	81%
At the time of discharge, healthcare follow-up instructions were clearly communicated to me:	80%
The hospital care team have been very helpful in explaining services I need following discharge:	73%
At discharge, the hospital staff answered all of my questions about follow-up care:	73%
I understand common side effects of my medications:	69%
I received clearly written healthcare follow-up instructions:	65%
The medication sheet I received at discharge was complete:	59%
The information I received at discharge has generally been very easy to understand:	40%

Note: Questions were reworded to report responses in the same direction

FIGURE 1. Incomplete Medication Sheet

Current Meds: Glyburide, Hytrin, Prednisone, Protonix, Trazodone, Zofran

Physician Satisfaction

Surveys were sent to more than 125 physicians. Forty-two physicians responded to the surveys; 43% were family practitioners and 36% gen-

FIGURE 2. Illegible Medication Sheet

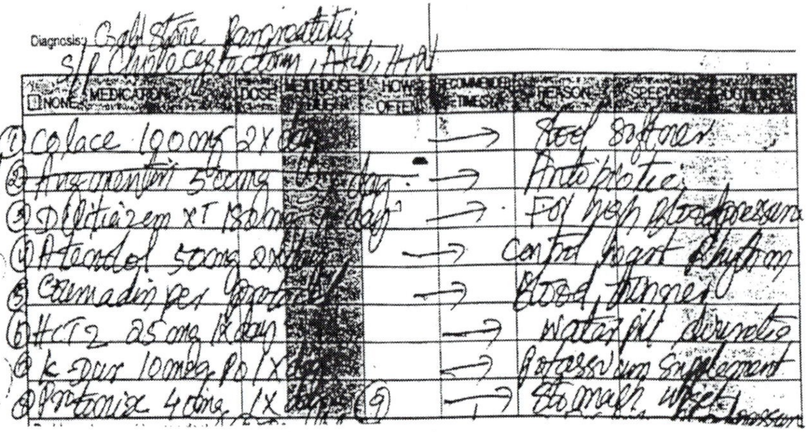

FIGURE 3. Medication Sheet with Medical Terminology and Missing Information

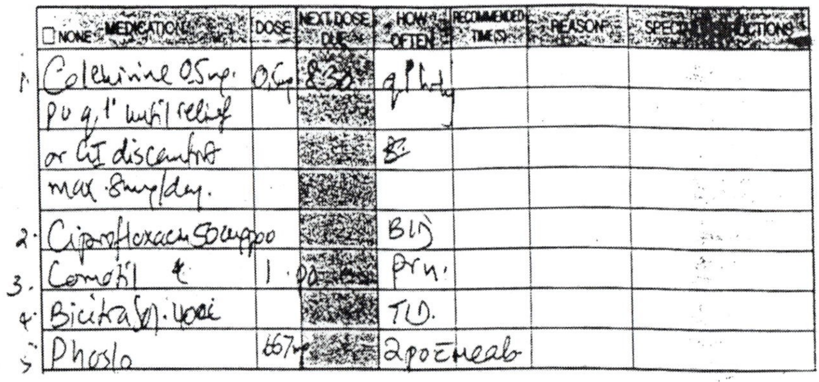

eral internists, with 21% subspecialists. More than two-thirds (69%) had combined office practices as well as admitting privileges, 19% had office practices only, and 12% were members of the inpatient rounding teams. Overall more than half (59%) of the physicians felt that the current system of communicating medications to patients and providers at hospital discharge was poor. No one rated any of the communications as excellent, and few identified them as "good." In terms of the condition of the completeness and legibility of the medication sheet, physicians were generally divided, although most (62%) agreed that patients have difficulty understanding the medications sheet and instructions. Most of the physicians agreed that they were aware of the medications taken by their patients at the time of hospital admission and that the medications listed on the medication sheet were accurate (see Table 2).

DISCUSSION

According to primary care physician reports, discharge medication records were not adequately or consistently being communicated to the primary care physician. Primary care physicians also felt that their patients were not clear as to what medications/doses they should be taking following hospital discharge. Interestingly, physicians' perceptions of the completeness of the medical record medication listings were more favorable than what was found in the chart review.

Physician and hospitalist general dissatisfaction with the process of gathering medications data from older hospitalized patients and accurately communicating these medications to patients, primary care physicians and other care settings upon hospital discharge, coupled with the data obtained from the chart review, led to the development of a proposal to organize a task force to address this issue. Funds were solicited and received from a source within the medical group to redesign the hospital process of documenting and communicating medications to older adults at hospital discharge.

A task force was convened to review the current medication communication processes at hospital discharge and make recommendations for changes. The task force consisted of hospitalists, primary care physicians, staff nurses, discharge planners, and pharmacists. A principal aim of the task force was to develop a method that allows the medication record to be printed rather than handwritten, using a database with drop down menus for medication selection. This process would reduce medication errors related to illegibility, misspellings, and use of medical terminology. Further, the electronic medication record would serve several needs. A copy of the medication record could be sent to the appropriate outpatient service the patient would be using (e.g., home health or Long Term Care), to the primary physician, and to the pharmacists to fill new medication orders prior to discharge. It was envisioned that this process would further reduce errors by eliminating multiple forms used to list medications and save staff time by eliminating duplicative efforts.

TABLE 2. Physician Satisfaction Survey

Question	Excellent	Good	Average	Poor	Very Poor
Upon discharge from the hospital, the communication I receive regarding my patients' medications and instructions are:	0%	16%	47%	18%	11%
Upon discharge from the hospital, the communications my patients receive regarding their medications and instructions are:	0%	18%	37%	37%	0%
Our current system of communicating discharge medications to patients, primary care physicians, and continuing care providers is:	0%	7%	33%	43%	17%
Outpatient Survey	Strongly Agree	Some-what Agree	Some-what Dis-agree	Strongly Dis-agree	Don't Know
The routine and PRN medications included on the medication sheet are incomplete	21	36	10	10	23%
The medication sheet my patients receive at discharge from the hospital is legible	26	33	15	5	21%
The medication sheet is an accurate list of the medications my patient should be taking	5	41	26	13	15%
My patients' have difficulty understanding the medications sheet and instructions	18	44	21	3	21%
Inpatient Survey	Strongly Agree	Some-what Agree	Some-what Disagree	Strongly Dis-agree	
At the time of admission, my patient has a clear understanding of correct medication to take	3	70	20	7	
At the time of admission, it's difficult for me to determine which medications the patient is currently taking	17	62	17	3	
Discharge medication instructions are written using language that my patients understand	14	57	25	4	
When completing discharge medications instructions, I am confident that the medications listed are correct and complete	21	43	25	11	

For six months, the task force met monthly to develop and test an electronic medications database and to develop new protocols for communicating medications to older patients at hospital discharge. A Microsoft Office Access-based electronic mediation sheet was developed and program shortcuts were loaded on computers throughout the medical center. Extensive training was conducted among all physicians, nurses, floor clerks, discharge planners, and emergency department clerks and nurses on the use of the electronic medication record. In addition, older patients with seven or more medications, patients at higher risk for medication error and duplication, or those admitted because of a medication error were to be referred to the hospital pharmacist who would review all medications and provide patient/family education on each prior to discharge.

Once in place, however, few physicians actually used the electronic discharge medication system. Reminder cards were posted on each computer and storyboards were developed and distributed throughout the medical center. Despite these efforts, transition from customary handwritten documentation of medications and discharge orders to the electronic form did not occur within the first six months of implementation. Pharmacist review for high-risk patients also was not routinely employed due to competing demands and pharmacy staffing changes.

In developing the electronic medication system, the complexity of the process of determining patients' proper drug list was elucidated. Our health care system contains many labor wasting steps, where multiple providers record the same information in multiple places; nurses complete a list of medications on a discharge instruction sheet, physicians write medication orders on a discharge summary, a discharge planner sends a list of medications to referral services such as home health or hospice. Not only does each provider duplicate actions of other providers, but also each step offers another potential point for a medication error through omission, commission or through other forms of documentation.

Additionally, each care setting represents another potential point for a medication change and therefore, a possible medication error. The lack of coordination and communication between care settings (Coleman, 2003) further exacerbates the ability to determine an accurate list of medications and dosages for hospitalized patients. In many instances, the physicians providing hospital care may only have seen the patient once or twice but were responsible for determining an accurate medication list, including those medications unrelated to the current hospitalization.

Identifying the appropriate medications is just the first step to comprehensive discharge process. The hospital care team must also work to ensure that the older patient and/or the caregiver are knowledgeable about the purpose of the drugs and how they are to be taken. These discussions must be followed by similar communications with the primary care physician and other medical professionals at the transfer care settings to further reduce redundancies and potential medication errors at these transfer settings.

Finally, simply developing a better communication system is not sufficient in addressing the problem. Measures must be taken to ensure that organizational policies are in place to support the introduction and adoption of new practices. In our situation, in the development of the electronic discharge medication record, key hospital physician leaders were present and part of the planning team. They engaged in pre-testing the electronic record and contributed to modifying it to increase ease of use. However, the project was not identified by administration as a required practice and therefore was viewed as an "optional" process, rather than a mandatory measure. Further, the project did not have sufficient resources to provide onsite, ongoing mentoring and support to aid the physicians and other clinical staff in the use of the system. Thus, the key barrier to implementation of the new form was our inability to change the practice patterns among the varied providers, despite their universal recognition of the extent of the problem and need for improved methods. In rolling out new medical care models, project champions/advocates are needed in addition to strong administrative leadership support for implementing the new process.

This small study clearly supports larger studies that have identified hospital discharge as a point of particular high risk of medication error for older adults (Beers, Munekata, & Storrie, 1990; Lau, Florax, Porsius, & De Boer, 2000; Beers et al., 1992). Additionally, although patients generally reported high levels of satisfaction with communication about medications and discharge orders, the written orders did not correlate with patient reports in terms of number of medications. This finding is consistent with others (Beers, Munekata, & Storrie, 1990; Lau, Florax, Porsius, & De Boer, 2000) who found that medications recorded in the hospital medical record are often times incomplete.

REFERENCES

Bates, D. W., Cullen, D. J., Laird, N., Peterson, L. A., Small, S. D., Servi, D. et al. (1995). Incidence of adverse drug events and potential adverse drug events: Implications for prevention. *JAMA, 274*(1), 29-34.

Beers, M. H. (2000-2001). Age-related changes as a risk factor for medication-related problems. *Generations, 24*(4), 22-27.

Beers, M. H., Munekata, M., & Storrie, M. (1990). The accuracy of medication histories in the hospital medical records of elderly persons. *J Am Geriatr Soc, 38*(11), 1183-1187.

Beers, M. H., Sliwkowski, J., & Brooks, J. (1992). Compliance with medication orders among the elderly after hospital discharge. *Hosp Formul, 27*(7), 720-724.

Boockvar, K., Fishman, E., Kyriacou, C. K., Monias, A., Gavi, S., & Cortes, T. (2004). Adverse events due to discontinuations in drug use and dose changes in patients transferred between acute and long-term care facilities. *Arch Intern Med, 164*(5), 545-550.

Coleman, E. A. (2003). Falling through the cracks: Challenges and opportunities for improving transitional care for persons with continuous complex care needs. *J Am Geriatr Soc, 51*(4), 549-555.

Hayes, K. S. (1999). Adding medications in the emergency department: Effect on knowledge of medications in older adults. *J Emerg Nurs, 25*(3), 178-182.

Hedges, J. R., Singal, B. M., Rousseau, E. W., Sanders, A. B., Bernstein, E., McNamara, R. M. et al. (1992). Geriatric patient emergency visits. Part II: Perceptions of visits by geriatric and younger patients. *Ann Emerg Med, 21*(7), 808-813.

Johnson, C. E., Christmas, C., & Dunne, M. (2004). High rate of errors on transfer dictations to subacute care. *J Am Geriatr Soc, 52*(1), S10.

Kahl, A. (1992). Geriatric education centers address medication issues affecting older adults. *Public Health Report, 107*, 37-47.

Kohn, L. T., Corrigan, J. M., & Donaldson, M. S. (1999). *Errors in health care: A leading cause of death and injury.* Washington, DC: Institute of Medicine.

Larsen, P. D., & Hoot Martin, J. L. (1999). Polypharmacy and elderly patients. *AORN Journal, 69*(3), 619, 621-622, 625, 627-628.

Lau, H. S., Florax, C., Porsius, A. J., & De Boer, A. (2000). The completeness of medication histories in hospital medical records of patients admitted to general internal medicine wards. *Br J Clin Pharmacol, 49*(6), 597-603.

Lazarou, J., Pomeranz, B. H., & Corey, P. N. (1998). Incidence of Adverse Drug Reactions in Hospitalized Patients: A Meta-Analysis of Prospective Studies. *JAMA, 279*(15), 1200-1205.

Lesar, T. S., Briceland, L., & Stein, D. S. (1997). Factors related to errors in medication prescribing. *JAMA, 277*(4), 312-317.

Paparella, S. (2004). Avoiding dangerous abbreviations and dose expressions. *J Emerg Nurs, 30*(1), 54-58.

Sobel, H., Medina-Walpole, A., & Katz, P. (2004). Information transfer between levels of care: A pilot study. *J Am Geriatr Soc, 52*(1), S97.

Medications Management in Older Persons: What Can Be Achieved in the International Community?

Lilian M. Azzopardi, BPharm, MPhil, PhD

SUMMARY. As the population ages worldwide, it is important to examine the challenges that are presented in the use of pharmaceutical treatments. This article comments on what is being done in the international community to promote rational use of medications and elimination of medication-related problems. Efforts are underway to identify elders at highest risk and to encourage communication and collaboration between the patient and the health care team, as well as collaboration among disciplines. Solutions to improve medication management are discussed, particularly those presented at a recent conference on Medication Management in Older Patients held under the ageis of the United Nations' International Institute on Ageing (INIA), Malta. These include evidence-based prescribing, interdisciplinary collaboration with increased clinical pharmacist involvement, and implementing programs that increase concordance between patient and health practitioner. Among the

Lilian M. Azzopardi is Senior Lecturer at the Department of Pharmacy, University of Malta.

Address correspondence to: Lilian M. Azzopardi, BPharm, MPhil, PhD, University of Malta, Department of Pharmacy, Msida, Malta.

[Haworth co-indexing entry note]: "Medications Management in Older Persons: What Can Be Achieved in the International Community?" Azzopardi, Lilian M. Co-published simultaneously in *Home Health Care Services Quarterly* (The Haworth Press, Inc.) Vol. 24, No. 1/2, 2005, pp. 137-146; and: *Improving Medication Management in Home Care: Issues and Solutions* (ed: Dennee Frey) The Haworth Press, Inc., 2005, pp. 137-146. Single or multiple copies of this article are available for a fee from The Haworth Document Delivery Service [1-800-HAWORTH, 9:00 a.m. - 5:00 p.m. (EST). E-mail address: docdelivery@haworthpress. com].

conference's conclusions is that more resources need to be allocated for medication management in the home arena. *[Article copies available for a fee from The Haworth Document Delivery Service: 1-800-HAWORTH. E-mail address: <docdelivery@haworthpress.com> Website: <http://www.HaworthPress. com> © 2005 by The Haworth Press, Inc. All rights reserved.]*

KEYWORDS. Medication management, older persons, evidence-based prescribing, interdisciplinary collaboration, concordance, pharmaceutical care, domiciliary services

As the worldwide population ages, it is important to examine the challenges that are presented when caring for older persons, particularly in the use of pharmaceutical treatment. Inappropriate drug use in older persons continues to be a primary area of concern as reported recently in the Archives of Internal Medicine which discusses findings of a study on outpatient elderly population (Australian Government Department of Health and Aging [DHA], 2004). The study reports the number of Beers list drugs, drugs that are associated with side effects in older persons and therefore should be avoided, prescribed to older persons in a one-year period. Throughout the year, more than 1 in 5 participants filled a prescription for a drug that should generally be avoided in elderly patients and almost 1 in 20 filled prescriptions for two or more of these drugs. Additional evidence exists documenting inappropriate drug prescribing in older persons. Fahey, Montgomery, Barnes, and Protheroe (2003) executed a study in the United Kingdom that revealed problems in medications management in terms of overuse of unnecessary or harmful drugs, under-use of beneficial drugs, and poor monitoring of chronic disease. Other medication-related challenges include rational drug use, patient education on drug therapy, compliance to drug therapy, and provision of seamless care. These challenges are experienced worldwide.

What is being done in the international community to promote the elimination of these medication-related problems? Efforts are underway to identify elders at highest risk and to encourage communication and collaboration between the patient and the health care team as well as collaboration among disciplines. Solutions for medication-related problems are being considered: education, communication, rational drug use, improved medication management, and cross-discipline healthcare team training beginning in the classroom and in early clinical experiences. And of course, adequate funding for these activities is essential for successful outcomes.

In 1982 the United Nations World Assembly on Aging was organized during which the *Vienna International Plan of Action on Aging* was established (United Nations, 2004). This action plan presents policy on aging and also includes a section on issues to be considered in the management of the health of older persons. The policy examines general issues such as social welfare and income security as well as health and nutrition. It was determined that care of older persons should not only be focused on disease diagnosis but should involve a holistic approach, taking into account physical, mental, social, spiritual and environmental factors. Systems should be established to sustain interdisciplinary care and specialized training, and specific standards should be developed for the provision of services to older persons.

In 1988 the International Institute on Ageing (INIA) in Malta, under the auspices of the United Nations, was established with the aim of providing multi-disciplinary education and training in specific areas related to aging. The issues, challenges and solutions discussed during a recent international conference sponsored by INIA are an apt way to summarize what health care professionals face worldwide and to offer some potential solutions and examples of successful programs that can be adopted.

In 2004, the INIA hosted a conference on Medication Management in Older Patients in Malta, collaborating with the European Society of Clinical Pharmacy (ESCP) the Special Interest Group (SIG) for Geriatrics and others. ESCP is an international association with an overall mission to develop and promote rational and appropriate use of medicines and medical devices by individuals and society. The SIG-Geriatrics is a group within ESCP with a special interest in research and projects regarding the care of older persons.

During this conference, a diverse group of health professionals from developing and developed countries engaged in a healthy discussion on what can be achieved in the medications management of older persons. Current trends in prescribing for older persons, pharmaceutical care issues for medication use in older persons, and care issues in older persons management were examined. The multidisciplinary background of faculty and participants provided an opportunity for various perspectives to be presented and for physicians, pharmacists and nurses to dialogue together in workshops addressing issues such as the prevention of falls and fractures, adherence to prescribed drug regimens, and disease management of patients with Parkinson's disease.

The conference plenary session presented by Cameron Swift, PhD, FRCP of the UK, began with the positive premise that aging and good health can co-exist, particularly now with the potential to change patients' health status into late life, to intervene and to modify with treatment as the evidence grows of the benefits of judiciously used medications. The goal for practitioners is to use evidence-based prescribing methods and to address issues of inappropriate prescribing more energetically.

Several key concepts presented by Dr. Swift on issues pertinent to drug use in older persons included:

- the value of evidence-based models to guide rational prescribing,
- the practice of pharmaco-vigilance to assess the effect of medications, i.e., the clinical results and risks in large populations including older persons and improved reporting to investigate the true incidence of adverse drug reactions, and
- interdisciplinary collaboration, particularly inclusion of the pharmacist on patient care teams. (This theme was echoed throughout other sessions, although other participating physicians cautioned that each health discipline should know their roles and boundaries.)

The importance of medication management and the necessitity of including medication review within comprehensive geriatric assessments were emphasized. The recommended method to provide this most efficiently is to add a drug review component to existing systems within patient care. For example, it is compulsory in a UK geriatric program for teams of pharmacists and prescribers to perform drug utilization review (DUR) audits together using evidence-based guidelines in the audit (Swift, 2004).

Another potential solution to inappropriate prescribing is the development of specific formularies and drug use protocols for the elderly. In a roundtable discussion on formularies and protocols, several examples were cited on the use of geriatric formularies in hospital to assist practitioners in choosing appropriate pre-discharge drugs. Some programs extend the formulary of drugs for older patient care to include protocols developed collaboratively with physicians and pharmacists for managing chronic conditions such as hypertension, diabetes, and constipation. Emphasis was made to include the participation of prescribing physicians in any process of drug formulary development, utilization and evaluation. Some participants suggested considering routine drug review in the absence of specific formularies.

The World Health Organization (WHO) Essential Drug List and its use were addressed in a debate led by Kees de Joncheere (2004), WHO Regional Director, Europe. In 1984 a World Health Organization Assembly resolution (WHA37.33) on the rational use of drugs requested "to continue to develop activities at national, regional and global levels aiming at the improvement of . . . prescription practices and the provision of unbiased and complete information about drugs to the health professions and to the public." Later resolutions (WHA47.13 and WHA49.14) reinforced this statement. WHO's "Policy Perspectives in Medicines: The Selection of Essential Medicines" (2002) provides an in-depth discussion on key policy issues, practical applications of the EM concept and key factors for successful implementation of an EM list.

Essential medicines (EM) are those that satisfy the priority health care needs of the population and the value of such a list is a global concept relevant to today's challenges, particularly with an increase in chronic disease in many parts of the world. The WHO Model List of Essential Medicines is both a model product and a model process concerning equal access to quality medication in an equitable process. The concept of selecting medicines is global, and should be applied according to each national situation. Many developed countries use the essential medicines concept but use different names, e.g., reimbursement list, positive list. De Joncheere stressed that the list is "a floor, not a ceiling" that strives to promote rational use of medicine: right drug for the right patient at the right dose given at the right time and advocates at the right price.

The selection of essential medicines, preferably linked to standard clinical guidelines, is a crucial step in ensuring access to health care and in promoting rational use by health professionals and consumers; however, there may be some challenges faced with aging populations. The elderly have special characteristics and needs due to their altered metabolism, frequent co-morbidity, and presence of polypharmacy, thus require special attention when prescribed medications. These characteristics require adaptation of dosages and drug review to minimize polypharmacy and the potential for drug-drug interactions and to improve adherence to the treatment plan. Furthermore, it is essential to improve therapeutic formulations and packaging to ensure the appropriate use of medication.

Other key points asserted by Kees de Joncheere included:

- How to improve prescribing when the rational use of medicines is not always easy to define? Appropriate use of medicines depends on rational prescribing and information. Whole and coherent system approaches are needed by establishing partnerships among all responsible participants, including health professionals and the patient; clinical pharmacologists and clinical pharmacists should be key participants.
- Because there are no easy or quick solutions, any change will require resources. No one approach can be effective in changing professional behaviour. Some suggestions to facilitate improvement include education, including academic detailing, support groups, newsletters, etc., implementation of formularies and treatment guidelines, careful budgeting and adequate IT support.

One of the most important final issues raised by de Joncheere was that once patients get their medications–either post hospital discharge or after visiting a practitioner, little is known about what happens at home. He advocates that more resources need to be allocated for medication management in the home arena (de Joncheere, 2004).

An example of enlightened government allocation for in-home services that came to light during the conference is found in Australia where the Department of Health and Aging has implemented an integrative service that utilizes an interdisciplinary and patient-focused approach to solving the medication crisis experienced in many healthcare settings today. Programs with this service had positive clinical results, and had a significant reduction in healthcare costs (DHA, 2004).

The author's own experience in Malta and that of others can serve to highlight some important themes to improve medication use raised during the conference. The role of pharmacist clinician as part of the healthcare team of older adults is worthy of consideration. In the 1989 *Drug Intelligence and Clinical Pharmacy Journal*, Mason states that "the pharmacist should be a drug therapy specialist as well as an information delivery specialist" (Mason, 1989). Interventions by pharmacists provide an opportunity to improve medication use in older persons by presenting information on the choice of drugs used for older persons, increasing patient knowledge on drug therapy and therefore helping to overcome the challenges presented in medication management in older persons. Such an intervention is very important in medication management programs intended for the elderly living in a variety of settings.

Programs that increase concordance between patient and health practitioner are key to overcoming challenges in compliance, patient education, and good practice. Concordance is used to denote the degree to which the patient and the health practitioner agree about the nature of the illness and the need for management and the relative risks and benefit of the proposed line of treatment. The patient and or caregiver's views are taken into account during the prescribing and other phases of treatment. Some strategies to improve adherence and reach concordance include pharmacist interventions to initiate and facilitate discussions with patients, elicit the patient's view and experience of treatment and provide information that meets one's needs, undertake routine medication review, liaise with other health professionals to ensure continuity of care and collaborate with prescribing physicians to identify treatment protocols.

Elderly patients, especially those living at home, may present with poor compliance or adherence for various reasons that range from confusion, fear of occurrence of side effects, to perceived costs and benefits of taking medications. By providing patient education and counseling on drug use, poor compliance may be minimized, and concordance reached.

An example of the provision of patient education by pharmacists and its impact on patient behavior is the practice in Malta at Zammit Clapp Hospital, an acute geriatric hospital. Pharmacists there provide a printed leaflet of the patient's discharge medication profile, which includes information on the use of the prescribed medications followed by a counseling session with the patient and their caregivers prior to discharge. This patient education intervention is intended to achieve seamless care and to reduce the problems with the transition of the patient from acute to primary care.

A prospective study was carried out at the hospital to evaluate this pharmacist intervention in counseling older patients upon discharge (Azzopardi, Serracino, Zarb, & Mizzi, 2003). Patient knowledge, their intended compliance and actual compliance on the use of medications prescribed after the counseling session and two weeks post-discharge was assessed. The results showed that patients' knowledge on the use of medications and intended compliance recorded was significantly higher after the counseling session. This indicates that the pharmacist counseling session reinforces patient knowledge and intention for compliance and adherence.

Another example of improving patient education is the government recommendation made in the United Kingdom in 1989 for patients to be supplied with written information about their medications before discharge from hospital (Green & Rees, 1999). These findings support the need for the provision of domiciliary services covering regular patient counseling and education of older persons who are living in the community. In the management of older persons in Europe, domiciliary care presents an opportunity to provide regular assistance to homebound patients. Pharmacists participating in medications management programs could act as navigators of older patient care by undertaking regular patient review and education while at the same time liaising with medical and health professional specialists covering the patients' medical conditions. Assistance which could be covered in the provision of domiciliary care services includes arrangement for repeat prescriptions to be ordered and delivered, assessment of patients' understanding on the use of their medications, patient counseling and discussion of drug-related problems, setting-up of compliance aids and ensuring accessibility to medications (including patient ability to open medication containers), and liaising with physicians and other health professionals.

In the United Kingdom, under the Care Standards Act 2000, national minimum standards (2002) were developed for care homes for older people. Under these standards, institutions for older persons are regulated and inspected. Among other factors, the standards cover documentation of patient care and medication distribution. The requirement for national minimum standards is also extending to the provision of domiciliary care services (Joshua, 2001; Allum, 2004).

Medication review is essential both for patients receiving home and community services as well as patients in residential homes. Multidisciplinary medication review of older patients can be time-consuming but is an advisable process for improving patient management as noted in the previously mentioned study funded by the Australian Department of Health. The Home Medicines Review (HMR) is a service that involves the collaborative work of General Practitioners (GPs) and pharmacists. At the request of the GP and with the consent of the patient, an HMR referral is made to a pharmacist who then schedules an appointment at the patient's home and convenience. The pharmacist then conducts a thorough assessment of the medications using clinical information provided from the GP. Once the assessment is complete, the pharmacist provides a review that includes suggested medication management strategies. Next the two professionals develop a written medication management plan, which is discussed with the patient.

Studies conducted in Australia have found that programs with this service improve patient satisfaction, understanding of and concordance with medication regimens, have positive clinical results, strengthen relationships between GP, patient and pharmacist and have a significant reduction in healthcare costs (DHA, 2004).

It is hoped that medication management programs for the care of older persons, whilst attempting to address the issues of patient education, compliance, rational and appropriate prescribing and seamless care, also embrace the concept of a multidisciplinary approach so as to achieve the goals in the most effective manner. In Malta we have the unique situation of the medical school and pharmacy school being together in one faculty and this promotes the establishment of very good relationships between pharmacists and physicians.

This reflection on what has been achieved and on the identified areas for improvement across the two continents supports Marshall McLuhan's concept of a global village (McLuhan, 1964). The world has become one village in terms of communication, and we can state that we are also witnessing universality in the issues raised in health care. Care of the older persons is a global issue and the progress made and goals identified are quite similar across the Atlantic and even throughout the world.

Hope abounds for these diverse activities and leaderships to continue to collaborate to provide the required impetus for individual practitioners or groups of practitioners to develop or continue their participation in medication management programs so as to achieve optimal care for older persons.

REFERENCES

Allum, L. (2004). National minimum standards in care homes: What role do pharmacists have? *Pharm J. 272*, 387-390.

Australian Government Department is Health and Aging. (2004, August 24). *Home Medicines Review (HMR) Guidelines*. Retrieved December 10, 2004 from http://www.health.gov.au/internet/wcms/publishing.nsf/Content/health-epc-dmmr.htm.

Azzopardi, L.M., Serracino, I. A., Zarb, A.M., & Mizzi, R. (2003, May). *Pharmacist intervention in counseling older patients*. Conference proceedings at the 4th ESCP Spring Conference on Clinical Pharmacy, Lisbon, Portugal.

De Joncheere, K. (2004, October). *The WHO Essential Drug List in developing countries is a barrier to good older patient care*. Paper presented at the meeting of the International Institute on Aging, United Nations, Malta.

Fahey, T., Montgomery, A.A., Barnes, J., & Protheroe, J. (2003). Quality of care for elderly residents in nursing homes and elderly people living at home: Controlled observational study. *British Medical Journal, 326*, 580.

Gottlieb, S. (2004). Inappropriate drug prescribing in elderly people is common. *British Medical Journal, 329*, 367.

Green, P., & Rees, L. (1999). Hospital discharge of elderly patients: Is seamless care achieved? *Pharmaceutical Jouranal. 263*, R35.

Joshua, A. (2001). Role for pharmacists in the National Care Standards Commission. *Pharmaceutical Journal. 266*, 834.

Mason, J.L. (1989). Pharmacy education and its impact on practice. *Drug Intell Clin Pharm. 23*, 259.

McLuhan, M. (1964). *Understanding media.* New York: McGraw-Hill.

Swift, C. (2004, October). *The age factor in the use of medicines.* Paper presented at the meeting of the International Institute on Aging, United Nations, Malta.

United Nations. (n.d.) *Vienna International Plan of Action on Ageing.* Retrieved on December 10, 2004 from www.un.org/esa/socdev/ageing/ageipaa.htm.

World Health Organization. (n.d.) *Policy Perspectives in Medicines: The Selection of Essential Medicines 2002.* Retrieved on December 10, 2004 from www.who.int/medicines/organization/ood/ood_annual_rep.shtml

Other collaborators included the Department of Pharmacy of the University of Malta, Zammit Clapp Hospital for the Aged, and the Maltese Ministry for Health, Elderly and Community Services. The author was conference Secretariat.

Index

BOOK ORDER FORM!

Order a copy of this book with this form or online at:
http://www.HaworthPress.com/store/product.asp?sku=5693

Improving Medication Management in Home Care
Issues and Solutions

___ in softbound at $22.95 ISBN-13: 978-0-7890-3053-5 / ISBN-10: 0-7890-3053-5.
___ in hardbound at $44.95 ISBN-13: 978-0-7890-3052-8 / ISBN-10: 0-7890-3052-7.

COST OF BOOKS _____

POSTAGE & HANDLING _____
US: $4.00 for first book & $1.50
for each additional book.
Outside US: $5.00 for first book
& $2.00 for each additional book.

SUBTOTAL _____

In Canada: add 7% GST. _____

STATE TAX _____
CA, IL, IN, MN, NJ, NY, OH, PA & SD residents
please add appropriate local sales tax.

FINAL TOTAL _____
If paying in Canadian funds, convert
using the current exchange rate,
UNESCO coupons welcome.

❑ **BILL ME LATER:**
Bill-me option is good on US/Canada/
Mexico orders only; not good to jobbers,
wholesalers, or subscription agencies.

❑ **Signature** _____

❑ **Payment Enclosed: $** _____

❑ **PLEASE CHARGE TO MY CREDIT CARD:**
❑ Visa ❑ MasterCard ❑ AmEx ❑ Discover
❑ Diner's Club ❑ Eurocard ❑ JCB

Account # _____

Exp Date _____

Signature _____
(Prices in US dollars and subject to change without notice.)

PLEASE PRINT ALL INFORMATION OR ATTACH YOUR BUSINESS CARD

Name

Address

City   State/Province   Zip/Postal Code

Country

Tel   Fax

E-Mail

May we use your e-mail address for confirmations and other types of information? ❑Yes ❑No We appreciate receiving
your e-mail address. Haworth would like to e-mail special discount offers to you, as a preferred customer.
We will never share, rent, or exchange your e-mail address. We regard such actions as an invasion of your privacy.

Order from your **local bookstore** or directly from
The Haworth Press, Inc. 10 Alice Street, Binghamton, New York 13904-1580 • USA
Call our toll-free number (1-800-429-6784) / Outside US/Canada: (607) 722-5857
Fax: 1-800-895-0582 / Outside US/Canada: (607) 771-0012
E-mail your order to us: orders@HaworthPress.com

For orders outside US and Canada, you may wish to order through your local
sales representative, distributor, or bookseller.
For information, see http://HaworthPress.com/distributors

(Discounts are available for individual orders in US and Canada only, not booksellers/distributors.)

The Haworth Press Inc.   **Please photocopy this form for your personal use.**
www.HaworthPress.com

BOF05

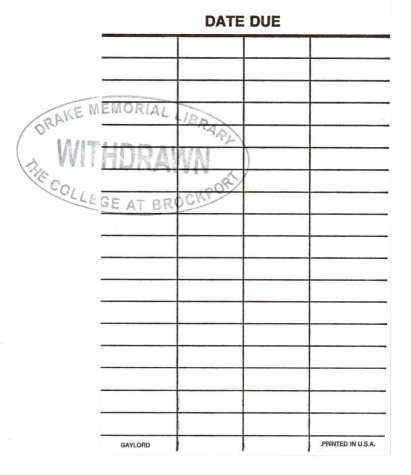